Englisches Konversations-Buch

für

Pharmazeuten.

Von

Dr. Th. D. Barry.

Dritte vermehrte und verbesserte Auflage,

herausgegeben von

Franz Capelle,
Besitzer von Dr. A. Sanders Adler-Apotheke in Norden.

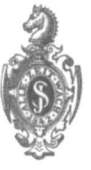

Berlin.
Verlag von Julius Springer.

ISBN 978-3-642-89279-0 ISBN 978-3-642-91135-4 (eBook)
DOI 10.1007/978-3-642-91135-4

Spamersche Buchdruckerei, Leipzig.

Vorwort.

Die vorliegende dritte Auflage des „Englischen Konversationsbuches" erscheint in erweiterter und übersichtlicher Anordnung und glaubt der Verfasser darin kurz zusammengefaßt zu haben, was dem Englisch lernenden Fachgenossen als unbedingtes Rüstzeug für Rezeptur und Handverkauf nötig ist. Die Hinzufügung der deutschen Aussprache englischer Worte ist in dieser neuen Ausgabe mit Bedacht fortgelassen worden, da das Erlernen derselben mündlichem Unterricht vorbehalten bleiben muß.

Der Umstand, daß eine dritte Auflage notwendig wurde, spricht für das Bedürfnis nach Büchern, welche dem mit Fremden-Publikum arbeitenden Apotheker Sprach- und Fachkenntnisse vermitteln, und hofft der Verfasser, daß das vorliegende Werkchen gleich den von Herrn Dr. Barry verfaßten ersten beiden Auflagen sich in Apothekerkreisen einer freundlichen Aufnahme erfreuen darf und dazu beiträgt, der vielfach gegebenen Anregung, sich fremdländische Fach- und Sprachkenntnisse anzueignen, gerecht zu werden.

Norden bei Norderney, Mai 1903.

Franz Capelle.

Inhalt.

		Seite
I.	Häufig vorkommende Ausdrücke im täglichen pharmazeutischen Leben	1
II.	Allgemeine Arzneimittel und dahin gehörende Ausdrücke	9
III.	Chirurgische und ähnliche Nebenverkaufsartikel der Apotheker	11
IV.	Der menschliche Körper und seine Teile	14
V.	Die Krankheiten des menschlichen Körpers	16
VI.	Die englische Nomenklatur	18
VII.	Drogen, Chemikalien, pharmazeutische Präparate	22
VIII.	Das englische Rezept	57
	1. Rezeptbeispiele aus der englischen Rezeptur	57
	2. Die englische Signatur	58
	a) Allgemeine Ausdrücke	58
	b) Beispiele englischer Signaturen	58
	c) Abkürzungen auf englischen Rezepten	59
IX.	Englische Gewichte, Hohl- und Längenmaße und ihre Beziehung zu den deutschen	61
X.	Münzsorten	63
XI.	Gespräche	63

I.

Häufig vorkommende Ausdrücke im täglichen pharmazeutischen Leben.

Abdampfen	to evaporate
Abdampfschalen	evaporating bassins
abgeben, eine Arznei	to dispense
abholen, - -	to fetch
abkochen	to boil
Abkochung	decoction
abkratzen	to scrape off
abkühlen	to cool
ablaufen	to run off
abliefern	to deliver
abmachen, z. B. ein Etikett	to take off a label
abmessen	to measure
abräumen	to clear away
abrechnen	to settle accounts
Abschrift eines Rezeptes	copy
abstauben	to dust
abteilen, z. B. Pulver	to divide in powders
abweichen, z. B. ein Etikett	to take off a label
abwiegen	to weight
anfertigen, eine Arznei	to make up a mixture
anfeuchten, ein Etikett	to moisten a label
anklopfen	to knock
anordnen	to order
anpreisen	to recommend
Anweisung	direction for use
anzünden, Feuer, Gas	to light te fire, gas
Apotheke	chemist's shop; chemist's and druggist's shop
- deutsche	german chemist's shop
- englische	english dispensary
- französische	french pharmacy
Apotheken-Besitzer	proprietor

Apotheken-Chef	governor
- =Eingang	entrance
- =Einrichtung	furniture
Apotheker	chemist, pharmaceutical chemist
- =Gehilfe	assistant
- =Lehrling	apprentice
Arznei	medicine
- =Mittel	remedy, physic, draught
- =Ware	drug
Arzt	physician, medical adviser, surgeon
auffüllen	to fill up
Aufguß	infusion
aufgießen	to infuse
aufkleben, ein Etikett	to label
aufräumen	to clear away
ausgießen	to empty
auspacken	to unpack
ausschreiben, eine Rechnung	to write an invoice
ausspülen	to clean
ausstreichen	to put out
Ballon	carboy
Becherglas	beaker
behandeln	to treat
Behandlung	treatment
bestauben	to make dusty
Beutel	bag
Bindfaden	string
bitter	bitter
blank	bright
Blatt, Blätter	leaf, leaves
Blattsilber	silver leaves
Blaustift	blue pencil
Bleifeder	pencil
Bleifolie	tinfoil
Bleistift	pencil
Blüte	flower
Boden	store
Dampf	steam
Dampfbad	water bath
dauern, kurze, lange Zeit	to take a short, long time
destillieren	to destill
Dienst	duty

Dienst haben	to be on duty
dienstfrei sein, heute abend	it is my night off
Docht	wick
Drahtnetz	wire gauze
Dreifuß	tripod
Duft	scent
durchlaufen	to run through
- langsam, schnell	to run slowly, quickly through the filter
- lassen	to filter
Eimer	bucket, pail
einnehmen	to take
einzunehmen	to be taken!
nicht einzunehmen	not to be taken!
einpacken	to make up a parcel
Einrichtung	furniture
einschreiben, ein Rezept	to enter a prescription
einweichen	to soak
einwickeln	to wrap up; to make up to a parcel
empfehlen	to recommend
engagieren	to engage
entleeren	to empty
entkorken	to draw the cork out
Etikett	label
etikettieren	to label
Exsiccator	desiccator
Faß	cask
Feder	pen
Federhalter	penholder
fein	fine
fertig sein	to be ready
fettig	greasy
feucht	moist
feucht werden	to moisten
Filter	filter
filtrieren	to filter
- langsam, schnell	to run slowly, quickly through the filter
Filtrierpapier	filter paper
Flasche	bottle, phial, flask
- ohne Teilstriche	plain bottle
- mit -	marked -
- von 6 Unzen Inhalt	six ounces bottle

Flasche klein, groß, mittel	bottle of small, large, medium size
- blaue	blue bottle
- eckige	square -
- enghalsige	bottle with a narrow neck
- große	big bottle
- kleine	small bottle
- leere	empty bottle
- mit Stöpsel	stoppered bottle
- weithalsige	wide mouthed bottle
Flüssigkeit	liquid
Gas	gas
- anzünden	to light the gas
- ausdrehen	to turn the gas out
- kleindrehen	tu turn the gas down
Gebrauchsanweisung	direction for use
Gehalt	salary
Gehilfe	assistant
gemessen	measured
gepulvert	powdered
Geruch	scent, smell
geruchlos	scentless
Geschmack	taste
geschmacklos	tasteless
Gewicht	weight
Gift	poison
- -Buch	- book
- -Flasche	- bottle
Glas	glass
- -Röhre	- tube
- -Stab	- stick
Glocke	bell
die Glocke ziehen	to ring the bell
grob	coarse
Handtuch	towel
Handverkauf	retail
Handverkaufstisch	retail counter
Handverkaufswage	scales
Hausapotheke	medicine case
Heilmittel	remedy
heiß	hot
herein!	come in!
Hofapotheker	chemist to the court

holen	to fetch
homöopathische Apotheke	homoeopatic chemist's shop
Infundierbüchse	infusion pot
infundieren	to infuse
Inhalt	contents
Kalt	cold
Keller	cellar
Kessel	boiler, kettle
Kiste	box
klar	clear
kleben	to stick; to paste
klebrig	sticky
kochen	to boil
kolieren	to strain
Kollege	fellow assistant
Kollatorium	strainer
kopieren	to copy
Kork	cork
– klein, mittel, groß	cork of small, medium, large size
– =Bohrer	corkborer
– =Zange	corkpress
– =Zieher	corkscrew
kündigen	to give notice to
Kupferkessel	copperkettle
Laboratorium	laboratory
Lackmuspapier	tasting paper
Laufbursche	boy, errand boy
lauwarm	tepid
Leder	leather
auf Leder streichen	to spread on leather
leer	empty
Lehre, Lehrzeit	apprenticeship
Lehrling	apprentice
leicht	light
Leinwand	linen
auf Leinen streichen	to spread on linen
liefern	to deliver
Löffel	spoon
– Dessert=	dessertspoon
– Eß=	tablespoon
– Thee=	teaspoon
Löschpapier	blotting paper

lösen	to dissolve
löslich	soluble
Maß	measure
Materialkammer	store room
Mensur	measure
Messer	knife
mischen	to mix
Mischung	mixture
Mörser	mortar
- aus Eisen	iron-mortar
- - Porzellan	porcelain-mortar
naß	wet
Oblaten	wafers, cachets
Ofen	stove
ordnen	to arrange
Ordnung	order
Paket	parcel
Papier	paper
Pergamentpapier	parchment paper
Pflaster	plaster
- streichen	to spread
Pillen	pills
- -Abschneider	pill knife
- -Brett	- tray
- -Glas	- glass
- -Maschine	- machine
- -Rollierer	- finisher
- -Schachtel	- box
- -Versilberer	- silverer
Pistill	pestle
Porzellanschale	porcelain dish
Pulver	powder
- fein, grob	- fine, coarse
- -Beutel	- bag
- -Kapsel	paper capsules
- -Schachtel	powder box
- - rund	- - round
- - viereckig	- - square
pulvern	to reduce to powder
putzen	to clean
Reagens-Gestell	test tube holder
- -Glas	test tube

Reagens-Papier	test paper
Rechnung	invoice
auf Rechnung von	on account of; o/a. o.
Regal	shelf
reiben	to triturate
rein	clean
reinigen	to clean
Rezept	prescription
- abgeben	to dispense a prescription
- anfertigen	to make up -
- aufschreiben	to write -
- kopieren	to copy -
- eintragen	to enter -
- wiederholen	to repeat -
Rezeptier-Pult	prescription desk
- -Tisch	- counter
riechen	to smell
- gut, schlecht	- good, badly
rot	red
Rotstift	red pencil
rühren	to stir
Saft	juice
Sägespäne	saw dust
Salbe	ointment
Salbentopf	ointment pot
- mit Deckel	covered ointment pot
Samen	seed
Schachtel	box
Schale	peel
Schaufenster	window
im Schaufenster auslegen	to put in the window
- - ausliegen haben	to have in the window
Schaukasten	show case
Scheidetrichter	separatory funnel
Schere	a pair of scissors
Schieblade	drawer
Schimmel	mould
schimmelig	mouldy
schimmeln	to get mouldy
schmecken	to taste
- gut, schlecht, leidlich	- nice, bad, pretty well
schmelzen	to melt
schmutzig	dusty
- werden	to get dusty

Schrank	chest
schwarz	black
schwer	heavy
Sieb	sieve
sieben	to sift
Siegellack	sealing wax
siegeln	to seal
Signatur	advice
signieren	to label
Spatel	spatula
spülen	to clean
Standgefäß	standard bottle
Stanniol	tinfoil
Stativ	support; retort stand
Stecknadeln	pins
Stempel	stamp
stempeln	to stamp
Suppositorien	suppositories
- -Form	suppositories' mould
süß	sweet
Tafelwage	counter balance
tektieren	to cap
Tekturpapier	caping paper
- blau, rot, gold, silber	blue, red, gold, silver
Tiegel	crucible
Tinktur	tincture
Trichter	funnel
trocken	dry
Trockenschrank	drying box
trocknen	to dry
tröpfeln	to drop
Tropfglas	droping bottle
trübe	cloudy
- werden	to get cloudy
Tür	door
- offen lassen	to let the door open
- schließen	to shut the door
- zu!	shut the door!
Überlaufen	to run over
Uhrglas	watch glass
umrühren	to stir
umschütteln	to shake
umschütteln!	shake the bottle!

nicht umschütteln!	not to be shaken!
umstürzen	to upset
unterschreiben, ein Rezept	to sign a prescription
Verreiben	to triturate
Versehen	mistake
- machen	to make a mistake
Wachs	wax
- -Kapseln	wax capsules
- -Papier	wax paper
Wage	balance
Waschbecken	washing basin
Wasserbad	water bath
Wasserbehälter	reservoir
weiß	white

II.

Allgemeine Arzneimittel und dahin gehörende Ausdrücke.

Abführmittel	purgatives
Abführ-Pastillen	aperient lozenges
- -Pillen	aperient pills
- -Trank	aperient draught, black draught
abführend wirken	to open the bowels, to act on the bowels
Verstopfung	constipation
verstopft sein	my bowels are not open
mild, stark, ziemlich stark	mild, strong, pretty strong
anregende Mittel	stimulating, inciting remedies
abgespannt, niedergeschlagen sein	to be down in spirit
Energielosigkeit, Mattigkeit	want of energy
ein vorzügliches Mittel für schwache Nerven	an excellent remedy for want of energy
Ätzmittel	caustics
Höllensteinstift	lunar caustic
auflösende Mittel	solvents
auflösen	to dissolve

Auflösung	lotion
(z. B. Borsäurelösung, Karbolwasser)	(boric acid, carbolic acid lotion)
Brechmittel	emetic
erbrechen, auswerfen	to vomit
sich erbrechen müssen	to be sick
Einpinselung	for rubbing on with a camel hair brush
Einreibung	embrocation
einreiben	to rub on, to smear on; to put on
Haareinreibung	hair lotion
Einspritzung	injection
einspritzen	to use as an injection
erweichende Mittel	emollients
Umschlag	cataplasme
Gurgelwasser	gargle
gurgeln	to gargle
ausspeien	to spit out
hinterschlucken	to swallow
Harntreibende Mittel	diuretics
Harn	urine
Untersuchung	analysis
untersuchen	to analyse
Heilmittel	remedy
Hühneraugenmittel	corn remedy
Hustenmittel	cough remedy
Husten-Mixtur	cough mixture
- -Pastillen	- lozenges
- -Tropfen	- drops
Latwerge	electuary, confection
Lösung	solution, lotion
Mischung	mixture
Öl	oil
Pastille	lozenge
Pflaster	plaster
Pflaster schmelzen	to melt a plaster
- streichen	to spread a plaster
- - auf Leder	- - - - up leather
- - - Leinen	- - - - up linen

Pille	pill
vergoldete Pille	gold coated pill
versilberte -	silver - -
verzuckerte -	sugar - -
Pulver	powder
pulvern	to reduce to powder
fein, grob	fine, coarse
Pulver machen	to prepare, to make up a powder
- einteilen	to divide in powders
- in Oblaten machen	to make up in cachets
Saft	juice
Salbe	ointment, salve
Salbe rühren	to stir an ointment
- schmelzen	to melt an ointment
Trank	draught
Abführtrank	black draught
Waschung	lotion
Augenwasser	eye lotion
Haarwasser	hair lotion
Mundwasser	mouth wash

III.
Chirurgische und ähnliche Nebenverkaufsartikel der Apotheker.

Augen-Douche	eye douche, eye cups
- Kappe	eye shade
- Tropfglas	eye tube, dropping tube
Beinlade	splint
Blutegelglas	leachtube
Brillen	spectacles
Bruchband	bruss
Brustsauger	breast glasses
Brust- und Lungenschutz	chest and lung protector
Brustwarzenhütchen	nipple shields
Charpie	lint

Einatmungsapparat	inhalers
Einnehme-Glas	medicine glass
- -Löffel	- spoon
Eisbeutel	icebag
Frottierhandschuhe	bathing gloves
Glas-Pinsel	glass brush
- -Spritze	- syringe
Glieder (künstliche)	artificial limbs
Gonorrhöebeutel	gonorrhoe bag
Gummiballonspritze	elastic ball syringe
Gummi-Finger	india rubber finger
- -Spritze	- - syringe
- -Strumpf	elastic stockings
- -Kniestrumpf	knee caps
Haar-Bürste	hairbrush
- -Nadeln	hairpins
Hals-Pinsel	throat brush
- -Schwamm	larynx sponge
Höllensteinstift	lunar caustic
Hühneraugen-Feile	cornfile
- -Messer	cornknife
Impfpockenschützer	vaccination shield
Impfstoff	vaccine lymph
Inhalationsapparat	throat inhalor
Irrigator	enema syringe
- -Gefäß	cystern
Kamm	comb
Katheter	catheter
Kehlkopfspiegel	laryngoscope
Kinder-Becher	feeding cups
- -Flasche	feeding bottle
- -Flaschenreiniger	- - brush
Klistierspritze	enemas
Luftkissen	air cushions
Lutscher	teat, india rubber teat
Monatsbinden	lady towels, diapers
Mutterrohr	tap
Nacht-Lampe	night lamp
- -Lichter	night lights

Nadel	needle
Nagelbürste	nailbrush
Nähseide	silk
Nasen-Douche	nose cups
- -Spritze	nose syringe
Ohren-Spritze	ear syringe
- -Reiniger	ear cleaner
Parfümzerstäuber	perfume sprinkler
Pinsel	camel hair brush
Pravazspritze	subcutaneous syringe
Puder-Beutel	powderbag
- -Quast	powderpuff
Pulvereinbläser	powderinsufflator
Rasierpinsel	shavingbrush
Respirator	respirator
Saugflasche	feeding bottle
Schlauch	india rubber tubing
Schminktopf	rouge pot
Schwamm	sponge
- -Beutel	spongebag
Spritze	syringe
Spritzkork	sprinkler stopper
Suspensorium	suspensory bandage
Thermometer	thermometer
Urinflasche	urine bottle
Verbandstoffe	dressing
Binde	bandage
Flanell-Binde	flannel bandage
Gaze- -	starched- -
Gips- -	water dressing bandage
Leinen- -	roll bandage
Mull- -	gauze -
Gaze	gauze
Jodoform-Gaze	jodoform gauze
Karbol- -	carbolic -
Sublimat- -	sublimat -
Lint	lint
Borlint	borlint
Watte	cotton wool
Karbol-Watte	carbolised cotton wool

Eisenchlorid-Watte	styptic cotton wool
Salicyl- -	salicylated - -
Sublimat- -	sublimat - -
Wärmflasche	hot water bag
Warzenhut	nipple shield
Zahn-Bürste	toothbrush
- -Stocher	toothpicks
Zungenreiniger	tongue scrape

IV.
Der menschliche Körper und seine Teile.

Achsel	armpits
Adern	veins
Arm	arm
den Arm brechen	to break the arm
ich habe den Arm gebrochen	my arm is broken
Auge	eye
angelaufenes Auge	blue eye
geschwollenes -	swollen eye
Augen-Brauen	eye brow
- -Lid	- lid
- -Wimpern	- lashes
Backe	cheek
Bein	leg
gebrochenes Bein	broken leg
geschwollenes -	swollen leg
Blut	blood
unreines Blut	bad blood
Brust	chest
Brustwarze	nipple
Daumen	thumb
Eingeweide	bowels
Ellenbogen	elbow
Ferse	heel
Finger	finger
sich den Finger ritzen	to scratch the finger
- - - schneiden	to cut - -

sich den Finger verbinden	to strap the finger
- - - verbrennen	to burn - -
Fuß, Füße	foot, feet
Fußgelenk	ankle
Galle	gall
Gesicht	face
Gesichtsfarbe	complexion
blaß	pale
blaß aussehen	to look pale
zart -	to have a delicate complexion
Glied	member
Haar	hair
hell, dunkel, schwarz	light, dark, black
dünn	thin
stark	thik
Ausgehen des Haares	to come off
stärken, das Haar	to make the hair grow
Hals	throat
Hand	hand
- =Fläche	palm of the hand
- =Gelenk	wrist
Haut	skin
empfindliche Haut	delicate skin
Herz	heart
Kehle	throat
Kinn	chin
Knie	knees
Knochen	bone
Knöchel	ankle
Körper	body
Kopf	head
Kahlkopf	bald head
Leber	liver
Lippe	lip
Lunge	lungs
Magen	stomach
Mandeln	tonsils
Nabel	navel
Nagel	nail
Nase	nose

Nasenlöcher	nostrils
Nerven	nerves
Nieren	kidneys
Ohr	ear
Rücken	back
Rückgrat	spine
Schädel	skull
Schläfe	temples
Schulter	shoulder
Sehnen	sinews
Stirn	forehead
Zahn, Zähne	tooth, teeth
Zahnfleisch	gums
Zehe	toe
Zunge	tongue

V.

Die Krankheiten des menschlichen Körpers.

Gesundheit	health
gesund	healthy
gesund sein	to be all right
Krankheit	illness
krank	ill
krank sein	to be ill

Ansteckung	contagion
Aufregung	excitement
aufgeregt sein	to be excited
Ausschlag	ecsceme
Bandwurm	tape worm
Bartflechte	beard ecsceme
Betrunkenheit	intoxication
betrunken sein	intoxicated, to be tipsy
Bleichsucht	chloriosis
bleichsüchtig sein	pale looking
Blutandrang	congestion

Blutfluß	hemorrhage
Blutverlust	loss of blood
Brandwunde	burn, scald
sich verbrennen	to burn
Daumengeschwür	thick (swollen) thumb
Drüsen	glands
Entzündung	inflammation
Erbrechen	vomiting
Erkältung	cold
sich erkälten	to catch a cold
Erschöpfung	exhaustion
erschöpft sein	to be exhausted
Erstickung	suffocation
Frostbeulen	chilblains
Frösteln	to shiver
Gelbsucht	jaundice
Geschwür	sore
Gesichtsschmerzen	pain in the face
Gicht	gout
Halsentzündung	sore throat
Heiserkeit	hoarseness
heiser sein	to be hoarse
Herzklopfen	beating heart
Hexenschuß	pain in the back
Hühneraugen	corns
Husten	cough
husten	to cough
jucken	to itch
kahl	bald
kahl sein	to have a bald head
Keuchhusten	wooping cough
Kopfweh	headache
- haben	to have a bad headache, to suffer from a bad headache
Leibschmerzen	pain in the bowels
Lungenentzündung	inflammation of the lungs
Magenschmerzen	pain in the stomach
niesen	to sneeze

Ohnmacht	fit
Ohrenschmerzen	pain in the ear
Quetschung	contusion
Schmerz	pain
schmerzhaft	painful
Schnupfen	cold
Schorf	scab
schwach	weak
Schweiß	perspiration
- treibend	sudorific
Schwindel	fainting, fit
Schwindsucht	consumption
schwitzen	to perspire
Sommerfleck	freckles
Tod	death
tot	dead
tödlich	deadly
Tripper	clap
Verstauchung	dislocation
Verstopfung	constipation
Warze	wart
Wunde	wound
wund sein	to be sore
Zahnschmerzen	toothache

VI.
Die englische Nomenklatur
ergibt sich aus folgenden Beispielen.

Acid	Säure
Acetic acid	Essigsäure
aromatic acid	aromatische Säure
concentrated acid	konzentrierte Säure
diluted acid	verdünnte Säure
Alcohol	Alkohol
absolute alcohol	absoluter Alkohol

Almond	Mandel
sweet almond	süße Mandel
Alum	Alaun
exsiccated alum	gebrannter Alaun
Ammonia	Ammonium
strong solution of Ammonia	Salmiakgeist
Antimony	Antimon
Antimony wine	Brechwein
Bark	Rinde
red Cinchona bark	Chinarinde
Beeswax	Wachs
white beeswax	weißes Wachs
Benzoas-Benzoate	benzoesaure Verbindungen
Ammonii Benzoas-Benzoate	benzoesaures Ammonium
Brandy	Franzbranntwein
Mixture of Brandy	- -Mixtur
Bromide	Bromid
Potassium Bromide	Bromkali
Bromine	Brom
Solution of Bromine	Bromwasser
Caustic	Ätzstift
toughened caustic	schwacher Höllensteinstift
Chalk	Kalk
prepared chalk	präparierter Kalk
Charcoal	Kohle
wood charcoal	Lindenkohle
Cloves	Nelken
infusiou of Cloves	Nelkenaufguß
Coal tar	Teer
Solution of coal tar	Teerwasser
Collodion	Kollodium
Blistering Collodion	Spanischfliegenkollodium
Confection	Latwerge
Confection of Roses	Rosenlatwerge
Ether	Äther
Acetic Ether	Essigäther
Extract	Auszug
alcoholic Extract of belladonna	alkoholischer Belladonnaextrakt
liquid Extract of Hydrastis	Hydrastisextrakt
green Extract of Hyoscyamus	frisches Bilsenkrautextrakt

Flowers	Blüten
Flowers of Sulfur	Schwefelblüten
Fruit	Frucht
Anise fruit	Anisfrucht
Galls	Galläpfel
Gall ointment	Galläpfelsalbe
Glycerin	Glycerin
Glycerin of boric acid	Borglycerin
Gum	Gummi
Mucilage of gum	Gummischleim
Honey	Honig
Borax Honey	Boraxhonig
Jodine	Jod
Jodine ointment	Jodsalbe
Iron	Eisen
Compound Mixture of Iron	zusammengesetzte Eisenmixtur
Juice	Saft
Juice of Lemon	Citronensaft
Lard	Schmalz
Benzoated lard	Benzoeschmalz
Lead	Blei
Lead acetate ointment	Bleisalbe
Leaves	Blätter
Bearberry leaves	Bärentraubenblätter
Lemon	Citrone
Syrup of Lemon	Citronensirup
Lime	Kalk
Lime water	Kalkwasser
Liniment	Liniment
Liniment of Ammonia	flüchtiges Liniment
Linseed	Leinsamen
Linseed oil	Leinöl
Lotion	Waschung
Black mercurial Lotion	schwarze Quecksilberwaschung
Lozenge	Pastille
Potassium chlorate Lozenge	Kalichloricumpastille
Male	Farn
liquid Extract of Male	Farnextrakt
Mercury	Quecksilber
Mercury pills	Quecksilberpillen

Milk	Milch
Milk of Sulfur	Schwefelmilch
Mixture	Mixtur
Castor oil mixture	Rizinusölmixtur
Mustard	Senf
volatile oil of mustard	ätherisches Senföl
Nutmeg	Muskatnuß
oil of Nutmeg	Muskatnußöl
Oil	Öl
Codliver oil	Lebertran
Ointment	Salbe
Boric acid ointment	Borsalbe
Peel	Fruchtschale
Orange peel	Pomeranzenschale
Peppermint	Pfefferminz
Peppermint water	Pfefferminzwasser
Pill	Pille
pill of lead and Opium	Bleiopiumpillen
pill of Quinine sulphate	Chininpillen
Pitch	Pech
Pitch plaster	Pechpflaster
Plaster	Pflaster
adhesive plaster	Heftpflaster
Poppy	Mohn
Syrup of poppy	Mohnsirup
Potash	Kalium
Bitartrate of Potash	doppelweinsaures Kali
Powder	Pulver
Compound powder of Ipecacuanha	Doversches Pulver
Resin	Harz
Scammony resin	Skammoniumharz
Root	Wurzel
Ipecacuanha root	Brechwurzel
Silver	Silber
Silver nitrate	salpetersaures Silber
Soap	Seife
Soap plaster	Seifenpflaster
Sodium	Natron
Bicarbonate of Sodium	doppelkohlensaures Natron

— 22 —

Solution	Lösung
Fowler's solution	Fowlersche Tropfen
Spirit	Spiritus
Spirit of Lavender	Lavendelspiritus
Squill	Meerzwiebel
Vinegar of squill	Meerzwiebelessig
Starch	Stärke
Glycerin of Starch	Glycerinstärke
Sulphur	Schwefel
sublimed sulphur	Schwefelblüten
Suppositories	Suppositorien
compound lead suppositories	zusammengesetzte Bleistuhl-zäpfchen
Syrup	Sirup
Syrup of phosphate of Iron	phosphorsaurer Eisensirup
Tablets	Tabletten
Nitroglycerine tablets	Nitroglycerintabletten
Tincture	Tinktur
Tincture of Opium	Opiumtinktur
Vinegar	Essig
Vinegar of Squill	Meerzwiebelessig
Water	Wasser
Chloroform water	Chloroformwasser
Wine	Wein
Quinine wine	Chinawein

VII.
Drogen, Chemikalien, pharmazeutische Präparate.

Absolute Alcohol	Alcohol absolutus (absoluter Alkohol)
Acetate of Morphine	Morphinae Acetas (essigsaures Morphium)
Acetate of Lead	Plumbi Acetas (essigsaures Blei)
Acetic acid.	Acid. acetic. (Essigsäure)
Acetic Ether	Aether acetic. (Essigäther)
Acid infusion of Cinchona	Infusum Cinchonae acidum (Chinarindenaufguß mit verdünnter Schwefelsäure)

— 23 —

Acid infusion of Roses	Infusum Rosae acid. (Rosen= aufguß mit verdünnter Schwefelsäure)
Acid solution of mercuric nitrate	Liquor Hydrargyri nitrat. ac. (salpetersaure Quecksilber= lösung)
Aconite root	Rad. Aconiti (Akonitwurzel)
Aconitine ointment	Ungt. Aconiti (Akonitsalbe)
Adhesive plaster	Empl. adhaes. (Heftpflaster)
Almond mixture	Mistura Amygdalae (Mandel= mixtur)
- oil	Ol. Amygdal. (Mandelöl)
Alum	Alumen (Alaun)
Ammoniacum and Mercury plaster	Empl. Ammoniaci et Hydrar- gyri (Ammoniakquecksilber= pflaster)
- mixture	Mistura Ammoniaci (Ammoniakharzmixtur)
Ammoniated Liniment of Camphor	Linimentum Camphor. ammon. (Kampferliniment)
- Mercury	Hydrargyr. praec. alb. (weißes Quecksilberpräzipitat)
- - ointment	Ungt. praec. alb. (weiße Queck= silbersalbe)
- Tincture of Ergot.	Tinctura Ergotae ammoniata (ammoniakalische Mutter= korntinktur)
- - - Gua- jacum	Tinctura Guajaci ammoniata (ammoniakalische Guajak= tinktur)
- - - Opium	Tinctura Opii ammoniata (ammoniakalische Opium= tinktur)
- - - Quinine	Tinctura Chinae ammoniata (ammoniakalische China= tinktur)
- - - Valerian	Tinctura Valerian. ammoniata (ammoniakalische Baldrian= tinktur)
Ammonium chloride of Mer- cury	Hydr. praec. alb. (weißes Quecksilberpräzipitat)
- Benzoate	Ammonium benz. (benzoesaures Ammonium)
- Bromide	Ammonium bromat. (Brom= ammonium)

Ammonium Phosphate	Ammonium phosphor. (phos= phorsaures Ammonium)
Amyl Nitrite	Amyl. nitros (Amylnitrit)
Anise Fruit	Fructus Anisi (Anissamen)
Anise Water	Aqua Anisi (Aniswasser)
Antimonial powder	Pulvis antimonialis (Anti= moniumpulver)
Antimonial Wine | Antimony Wine |	Vinum stibiatum (Brechwein)
Araroba powder	Araroba (Chrysarobin)
Argenti Nitras	Argent. nitr. (Höllenstein)
Arnica Rhizome	Rad. Arnicae (Arnikawurzel)
Aromatic powder of Chalk	Pulvis Cretae aromaticus (aromatisches Kalkpulver)
- - - - with Opium	Pulv. Cret. ar. c. opio (aro= matisches Kalkpulver mit Opium)
- Spirit of Ammonia	Spiritus Ammoniae aromaticus (aromatischer Ammoniak= spiritus)
- sulfuric acid	Ac. sulf. arom. (aromatische Schwefelsäure)
- Syrup	Syrup. aromaticus (aroma= tischer Sirup)
- - of Cascara	Syrup. Cascarae aromaticus (aromatischer Cascarasirup)
Arsenical Solution	Liquor arsenicalis (Fowlersche Tropfen)
Arsenious acid	Acid. arsenicosum (arsenige Säure)
Atropine ointment	Ungt. Atropinae (Atropinsalbe)
Balsam of Peru	Balsam. peruv. (Perubalsam)
- - Tolu	- tolutan. (Tolubalsam)
Bearberry leaves	Folia Uvae Ursi (Bären= traubenblätter)
Beeswax, white, yellow	Cera alba, flava (weißes, gelbes Wachs)
Belladonna leaves	Folia Belladonnae (Bella= donnablätter)
- root	Radix Belladonnae (Bella= donnawurzel)
- ointment	Ungt. Belladonnae (Bella= donnasalbe)
- plaster	Emplastrum Belladonnae (Belladonnapflaster)

Belladonna suppositories	Suppositoria Belladonnae (Belladonnastuhlzäpfchen)
Benzoated lard	Adeps benzoatus (Benzoeschmalz)
Benzoic acid	Acid. benzoic. (Benzoesäure)
- lozenge	Trochiscus acidi benzoici (Benzoetabletten)
Biborate of Sodium	Borax (Natriumbiborat)
Bichloride of Mercury	Hydrargyri perchloridum (Sublimat)
Bijodide - -	Hydrargyri jodidum rubrum (rotes Quecksilberoxyd)
Bismuth oxycarbonate	Bismuthi carbonas (kohlensaures Wismut)
- oxyde	Bismuth oxidum (Wismutoxyd)
- salicylate	Bismuthi salicylas (salicylsaures Wismut)
- oxynitrate	Bismuthi subnitras, Bismuth subnitric. (salpetersaures Wismut)
Bitartrate of Potassium	Potassii Tartras acidus (doppelweinsaures Kali)
Bitter Almond	Amygdala amara (bittere Mandel)
- - oil	Ol. Amygd. amar. (bitteres Mandelöl)
Bitter Orange peel fresh	Cort. Aurantii recens (frische Orangenschale)
- - - dried	Cort. Aurant. sicc. (trockene Orangenschale)
Black Draught	Mistura Sennae comp. (Wiener Trank)
- Mercurial Lotion	Lotio Hydrargyri nigra (schwache Quecksilberlösung)
- mustard seed	Sinapis nigrae semina (schwarzer Senf)
- Wash	Lotio Hydrargyri nigra (schwache Quecksilberlösung)
Blistering Collodion	Collodium vesiccans (blasenziehendes Kollodium)
- Liquid	Liquor epispasticus
Blue pill	Pilula Hydrargyri (abführende Quecksilberpillen)
Boracic acid	Acidum boricum (Borsäure)
Borax Honey	Mel boracis (Boraxhonig)

Boric acid ointment	Ungt. acid. borici (Borsalbe)
Broom Tops	Scoparii cucumina (Ginster)
Buchu leaves	Folia Buchu (Buchublätter)
Burgundy Pitch	Pix burgundica (Burgunderpech)
Caffeine	Caffeina (Koffein)
Calabar beans	Semina Physostigmatis (Kalabarbohnen)
Calomel ointment	Ungt. Hydrargyri subchlor. (Kalomelsalbe)
- pill compound	Pilula Hydrargyri subchloridi compos. (zusammengesetzte Kalomelpille)
Calumba root	Radix Calumbae (Colombowurzel)
Calx	Calcaria (Kalk)
Camphor water	Aqua Camphorae (Kampferwasser)
Camphorated oil	Linimentum Camphorae (Kampferliniment)
Cantharides ointment	Ungt. Cantharidis (Kantharidensalbe)
- plaster	Empl. Cantharidum (spanisch-Fliegenpflaster)
Capsicum ointment	Ungt. Capsici (spanisch-Pfeffersalbe)
Carawey fruit	Fructus Carvi (Kümmel)
- water	Aqua Carvi (Kümmelwasser)
Carbolic acid	Acid. carbol. (Karbolsäure)
- - lozenge	Trochiscus acidi carbolici (Karbolsäurepastillen)
- - ointment	Ungt. acid. carbolici (Karbolsäuresalbe)
- - suppositories	Suppositoria acidi carbolici (Karbolsäuresuppositorien)
Cardamom seeds	Fructus Cardamomi (Kardamom)
Cassia pulp	Pulpa Cassiae (Kassiamus)
Castor oil	Ol. Ricini (Rizinusöl)
- - mixture	Mistura olei ricini (Rizinusölmixtur)
Catechu lozenge	Katechupastille
Caustic Potash	Potassa caustica (Ätzkali)

Cerium Oxalate	Cerium oxalicum (oxalsaures Cerium)
Chalk prepared	Creta praeparata (präparierter Kalk)
- with mercury	Hydrargyrum cum Creta (präparierter Kalk mit Quecksilber)
- mixture	Mistura Cretae (Kalkmixtur)
Chamomile flowers	Flores Chamomillae (Kamillen)
Charcoal	Carbo ligni (Lindenkohle)
Cherry laurel leaves	Folia laurocerasi (Kirschlorbeerblätter)
- - water	Aqua laurocerasi (Kirschlorbeerwasser)
Chloral Hydras v. Hydrate	Chloralum hydratum (Chloralhydrat)
Chloric Ether	Spiritus Chloroformi (Chloroformspiritus)
Chlorinated lime	Calcaria chlorata (Chlorkalk)
- solution of lime	Liquor Calcis chlorinatae (Chlorkalklösung)
Chloroform water	Aqua Chloroformi (Chloroformwasser)
Chromic acid	Acidum chromicum (Chromsäure)
Chrysarobin	Araroba (Goapulver)
- ointment	Ungt. Chrysarobini (Chrysarobinsalbe)
Cinchona bark	Cortex Chinae (Chinarinde)
Cinnamom bark	- Cinnamomi (Zimt)
- water	Aqua Cinnamomi (Zimtwasser)
Citric acid	Acid. citricum. (Citronensäure)
Clarified Honey	Mel depurat (Honig)
Cloves	Caryophylli (Nelken)
Coal tar	Pix (Teer)
Coca leaves	Folia Cocae (Kokablätter)
Cocaine ointment	Ungt. Cocainae (Kokainsalbe)
Cochineal	Coccionella (Cochenille)
Codliveroil	Ol. Jecoris Aselli (Lebertran)
Colchicum corm	Colchici cormus (Herbstzeitlose)
- wine	Vinum Colchici (Colchicumwein)
- seeds	Semen Colchici (Colchicumsamen)
Collodion	Collodium (Kollodium)
- flexible	- elasticum (elastisches Kollodium)

Colocynth pulp	Pulpa Colocynthidis (Koloquintenmus)
Compound Bismuth lozenge	Trochiscus Bismuthii compos. (zusammengesetzte Wismutpastille)
Compound Calomel pill	Pilula Hydr. subchlor. comp. (zusammenges. Kalomelpille)
- Decoction of Aloes	Decoctum Aloes composit. (zusammengesetzte Aloeabkochung)
- Extract of Colocynth	Extr. Colocynthidis comp. (zusammengesetzter Koloquintenextrakt)
- infusion of Gentian	Infusum Gentianae comp. (zusammengesetzter Enzianaufguß)
- - - orange peel	Inf. cort. Aurantii cp. (zusammengesetzter Orangenaufguß)
- lead suppositories	Suppositoria plumbi cp. (zusammengesetzte Bleistuhlzäpfchen)
- liniment of Camphor	Liniment. Camphor ammoniat. (zusammengesetztes Kampferliniment)
- Mercury ointment	Ungt. Hydrarg cp. (zusammengesetzte Quecksilbersalbe)
- Mixture of Iron	Mistura ferri cp. (zusammengesetzte Eisenmixtur)
- - - Senna	Mistura Sennae cp. (zusammengesetzte Sennamixtur)
- pill of Asa foetida	pilula Asae foet. cp. (Stinkasantpille)
- - - Colocynth	- Colocynth cp. (zusammengesetzte Koloquintenpille)
- - - Galbanum	pilul. Galbani cp. (zusammengesetzte Galbanumpille)
- - - Gamboge	pilul. Cambogiae cp. (zusammengesetzte Cambogiapille)
- - - Mercurous chloride	pil. Hydr. subchlor. cp. (zusammengesetzte Kalomelpille)
- - - Soap	pilul. sapon cp. (zusammengesetzte Seifenpille)
- powder of Almonds	Pulv. Amygd. cp. (zusammengesetztes Mandelpulver)
- - - Catechu	Pulv. Catechu cp. (zusammengesetztes Catechupulver)

Compound powder of Cinnamom	Pulv. Cinnamomi cp. (zusammengesetztes Zimtpulver)
- - - Elaterin	Pulv. Elaterini cp. (zusammengesetztes Elaterinpulver)
- - - Ipecacuanha	Pulv. Ipecac. cp. (Doversches Pulver)
Compound powder of Jalep	Pulv. Jalapae cp. (zusammengesetztes Jalapenpulver)
- - - Kino	Pulv. Kino cp. (Kinopulver)
- - - Liquorice	- Glycyrrhizae cp. (Brustpulver)
- - - Opium	- Opii cp. (zusammengesetztes Opiumpulver)
- - - Rhubarb	- Rhei cp. (Rhabarberpulver)
- - - Scammony	- Scammon. cp. (zusammengesetztes Scammoniumpulver)
- - - Tragacanth	- Tragacanthae cp. (zusammengesetztes Tragantpulver)
- Rhubarb pill	pil. Rhei cp. (zusammengesetzte Rhabarberpille)
- Scammony pill	pil. Scammonii cp. (zusammengesetzte Scammoniumpille)
- Spirit of Ether	Spirit. Aetheris cp. (zusammengesetzte Hoffmannstropfen)
- - - Horseradish	Spiritus Armoraciae comp. (zusammengesetzter Meerrettichspiritus)
- Squill pill	pilula Scillae cp. (zusammengesetzte Meerzwiebelpille)
- Tincture of Benzoin	Tinct. Benz. cp. (zusammengesetzte Benzoetinktur)
- - - Camphor	Tinct. Camph. cp. (zusammengesetzte Kampfertinktur)
- - - Cardamoms	Tinct. Card. cp. (zusammengesetzte Kardamomtinktur)
- - - Chloroform and Morphine	Tinct. Chloroformi et Morphini (zusammengesetzte Chloroform- u. Morphiumtinktur)
- Tincture of Cinchona	Tinct. Chinae cp. (zusammengesetzte Chinatinktur)
- - - Gentian	Tinct. Gentian. (zusammengesetzte Enziantinktur)

Compound Tincture of Lavender	Tinctura Lavendulae comp. (zusammengesetzte Lavendeltinktur)
- - of Rhubarb	Tinct. Rhei cp. (zusammengesetzte Rhabarbertinktur)
- - of Senna	Tinct. Sennae cp. (zusammengesetzte Sennatinktur)
Concentrated phosphoric acid	Acid. phosph. con. (konzentrierte Phosphorsäure)
- solution of Columba	Liquor Columbae (konzentrierter Colombowurzelauszug)
- - - Chiretta	Liqu. Chirattae conc. (konzentrierter Chirettaauszug)
- - - Cusparia	Liqu. Cuspariae con. (konzentrierter Cuspariarindenauszug)
- - - Krameria	Liquor Krameriae conc. (konzentrierter Ratanhawurzelauszug)
- - - Quassia	Liq. Quassiae conc. (konzentrierter Quassiaholzauszug)
- - - Rhubarb	Liqu. Rhei cp. (konzentrierter Rhabarberwurzelauszug)
- compound solution of Sassaparilla	Liquor Sassae comp. conc. (zusammengesetzterSassaparillewurzelauszug)
- solution of Senega	Liquor Senegae conc. (konzentrierter Senegawurzelauszug)
- - - Senna	Liquor Sennae conc. (konzentrierter Sennesblätterauszug)
- - - Serpentary	Liq. Serpentariae conc. (konzentrierter Schlangenwurzelauszug)
Confection of Pepper	Confectio Piperis (Pfefferlatwerge)
- - Roses	- Rosarum (Rosenlatwerge)
- - Senna	- Sennae (Sennesblätterlatwerge)
- - Sulphur	- Sulfuris (Schwefellatwerge)
Conium fruit	Fructus Conii (Schierlingsfrucht)
- leaves	Folia Conii (Schierlingsblätter)

Conium ointment	Ungt Conii (Schierlingsſalbe)
Copaiba	Balsam Copaivae (Kopaiva-balſam)
Copper	Cuprum (Kupfer)
- sulphate	Cupr. sulfur. (ſchwefelſaures Kupfer)
Coriander fruit	Fructus Coriandri (Korianderſamen)
Corrosive Sublimate	Hydrargyri perchloridum (Sublimat)
Cotton wool	Gossypium (Watte)
Cream of Tartrar	Tartarus dep. (Cremor Tartari)
Creosote	Creosotum (Kreoſot)
- Mixcture	Mistura Creosoti (Kreoſotmixtur)
- Ointment	Ungt. Creosoti (Kreoſotſalbe)
Croton oil	Oleum Crotonis (Krotonöl)
Crushed linseed	Linum contusum (Leinſamenmehl)
Cubebs	Cubebae fructus (Cubeben)
Cupric Sulphate	Cupri sulphur (ſchwefelſaures Kupfer)
Curd Soap	Sapo purus (mediziniſche Seife)
Decoction of Logwood	Decoctum Haematoxyli (Kampecheholzabkochung)
- - Pomegranate bark	Decoctum Granati corticis (Granatrindenabkochung)
Digitalis leaves	folia Digitalis (Fingerhutblätter)
Dill fruit	Fructus Anethi (Dillſamen)
- water	Aqua Anethi (Dillwaſſer)
Diluted acetic acid	Acid. acetic dil. (verdünnte Eſſigſäure)
- Alcohol	Spiritus dilutus (verdünnter Spiritus).
- hydrobromic acid	Acid. hydrobromic. dil. (verdünnte Bromſäure)
- hydrochloric acid	Acid. hydrochlor. dil. (verdünnte Salzſäure)
- hydrocyanic acid	Acid. hydrocyanic. dil. (verdünnte Blauſäure)
- mercuric nitrate ointment	Ungt. Hydrargyri nitrati dilutum (ſchwache Queckſilbernitratſalbe)

Diluted Nitric acid	Acid. nitric. dil. (verdünnte Salpetersäure)
- nitro hydrochloric acid	Acidum nitro hydrochloricum dilutum (verdünnte Salpeter-Salzsäure)
- phosphoric acid	Acid. phosphor. dil. (verdünnte Phosphorsäure)
- solution of lead acetate	Liquor Plumbi subacetatis dilutus (Bleiwasser)
- sulphuric acid	Acid. sulf. dil. (verdünnte Schwefelsäure)
Discs	Lamellae (Gelatineplättchen)
- of Atropine	- Atropinae (Atropinlamellen)
- - Cocaine	- Cocainae (Cocainlamellen)
- - Homatropine	- Homatropinae (Homatropinlamellen)
- - Physostigmine	- Physostigminae (Physostigminlamellen)
Dover's Powder	Pulv. Ipecacuanhae comp. (Dover'sches Pulver)
Dried Alum	Alumen exsiccatum (gebrannter Alaun)
- ferrous Sulphate	Ferri Sulphas exsiccatus (getrocknetes Ferrosulfat)
- Sodium Carbonate	Sodii Carbonas exsiccatus (getrocknetes Natriumkarbonat)
Dry Extract of Euonymus	Extractum Euonymi sicc. (trockenes Evonyminextrakt)
- Thyroid	Thyroideum siccum (Thyreoidin)
East Indian Senna	Folia Sennae (Sennesblätter)
Effervescent Caffeine Citrate	Caffeinae Citras effervescens (brausendes Coffeincitrat)
- Epsom salt	Magnesii Sulphas effervescens (brausendes Bittersalz)
- Lithium Citrate	Lithii Citras effervescens (brausendes Lithiumcitrat)
- Magnesium Sulphate	Magnesii Sulphas effervescens (brausendes Bittersalz)
- Sodium Citrotartrate	Sodii citro-tartras effervescens (brausendes citronen-weinsaures Natron)

Effervescent Sodium Phosphate	Sodii Phosphas effervescens (brausendes Natriumphosphat)
- Sodium Sulphate	Sodii Sulphas effervescens (brausendes Glaubersalz)
- tartareted Soda powder	Pulvis Sodae tartaratae effervescens (brausendes weinsaures Sodapulver, Seidlitzpulver)
Effervescing Citrotartrate	Sodii Citrotartras effervescens (brausendes citronensaures Natron)
Elder flower	Sambuci Flores (Hollunderblüten)
- - water	Aqua Sambuci (Hollunderblütenwasser)
Elixir of Vitriol	Acidum sulfuricum aromaticum (aromatische Schwefelsäure)
Epsom salt	Magnesii Sulphas (schwefelsaure Magnesia)
Ergot	Ergota (Mutterkorn)
Eserine sulphate	Physotigminae Sulphas (schwefelsaures Eserin)
Ether	Aether (Äther)
Ethereal tincture of Lobelia	Tinctura Lobeliae aetherea (ätherische Lobelintinktur)
Eucalyptus Lozenge	Trochiscus Eucalypti gummi (Eucalyptusbonbon)
- Oil	Oleum Eucalypti (Eucalyptusöl)
- Ointment	Ungt. Eucalypti (Eucalyptussalbe)
Euonymus bark	Euonymi Cortex (Euonyminrinde)
Exsiccated Alum	Alumen exsiccatum (gebrannter Alaun)
- Ferrous Sulphate	Ferri Sulphas exsiccatus (trockenes Ferrosulfat)
- Sodium Carbonate	Sodii Carbonas exsiccatus (trockenes Sodapulver)
Extract of Barbados Aloes	Extractum Aloes barbadensis (Aloeextrakt)
- - Calabar been	Extr. Physostigmatis (Calabarbohnenextrakt)

Extract of Cascara Sagrada	Extractum Cascarae sagradae (Cascaraextrakt)
- - Chamomile	- Anthemidis (Kamillenextrakt)
- - Colchicum	- Colchici (Herbstzeitlosenextrat)
Extract of Ergot	Extractum Ergotae (Mutterkornextrakt)
- - Gentian	- Gentianae (Enzianextrakt)
- - Indian Hemp	- Cannabis Indicae (indischer Hanfextrakt)
- - Jalap	- Jalapae (Jalapenwurzelextrakt)
- - Krameria	- Krameriae (Ratanhiawurzelextrakt)
- - Liquorice	- Glycyrrhizae (Süßholzextrakt)
- - Nux vomica	- nucis vomicae (Brechnußextrakt)
- - Opium	- Opii (Opiumextrakt)
- - Rhubarb	- Rhei (Rhabarberextrakt)
- - Stramonium	- Stramonii (Stechapfelextrakt)
- - Strophantus	- Strophanti (Strophantusextrakt)
- - Taraxacum	- Taraxaci (Löwenzahnwurzelextrakt)
Fetid spirit of Ammonia	Spiritus Ammoniae fetidus (stinkender Ammoniumspiritus)
Fennel fruit	Fructus Foeniculi (Fenchel)
- water	Aqua Foeniculi (Fenchelwasser)
Ferrous sulphate	Ferri Sulphas, Ferrum sulfur. (schwefelsaures Eisen)
Figo	Ficus (Feige)
Flexible Collodion	Collodium flexile (elastisches Kollodium)
Flowers of Sulphur	Flores Sulphuris (Schwefelblüten)
Fluid Magnesia	Liquor. Magnesii carbonatis (flüssige kohlensaure Magnesia)

— 35 —

Fowler's solution	Liquor. arsenicalis (Arsenik= tropfen)
Foxglove	Folia Digitalis (Fingerhut= blätter)
Frankincense	Thus americanum (Harz von pinus palustris)
Friars balsam	Tinctura Benzoini comp. (zu= sammengesetzte Benzoe= tinktur)
Gallic acid	Acid. gallicum (Gallsäure)
Gall ointment	Ungt. Gallae (Gallsalbe)
- and Opium ointment	- - cum Opio (Gall= äpfelsalbe mit Opium)
Galls	Gallae (Galläpfel)
Gamboge	Cambogia (Cambogiaharz)
Gelsemium root	Radix Gelsemii (Gelsemium= wurzel)
Gentian root	- Gentianae (Enzian= wurzel)
Ginger	Rhizoma Zingiberis (Ingwer= wurzel)
Glacial acetic acid	Acid. acet. glaciale (Eisessig= säure)
Glucusimide | Gluside |	Glusidum (Saccharin)
Glycerin of Alum	Glycerinum Aluminis (Alaun= glyzerin)
- - Borax	- Boracis (Borax= glyzerin)
- - Boric acid	- acid. borici (Bor= säureglyzerin)
- - Lead subacetate	- Plumb. subaceta- tis (Bleizuckerglyzerin)
- - Pepsin	Glycerinum Pepsini (Pepsin= glyzerin)
- - Phenol	- acidi carbolici (Karbolsäureglyzerin)
- - Starch	Glycerinum amyli (Stärke= glyzerin)
- suppositories	Suppositoria Glycerini (Gly= zerinstuhlzäpfchen)
- of Tannic acid	Glycerinum acidi tannici (Gerbsäureglyzerin)
- - Tragacanth	- Traganthae (Tra= ganthglyzerin)

3*

Goa powder	Araroba (Chrysarobin)
Goulard's Extract	Liq. Plumb. subac. (Bleiessig)
- Lotion - Water	Aqu. Plumbi (Bleiwasser)
Green Extract of Belladonna	Extract. Bellad. viride (grünes [frisches] Belladonnaextrakt)
- - - Hyoscyamus	Extract. Hyoscyami (Bilsenkrautextrakt)
Gregory's powder	Pulvis Rhei comp. (zusammengesetztes Rhabarberpulver)
Grey's powder	Hydrargyrum cum Creta (Quecksilberkalkpulver)
Guajacum resin	Resina Guajaci (Guajakharz)
- Lozenge	Trochiscus Guajaci (Guajakpastille)
- mixture	Mixtura Guajaci (Guajakmixtur)
- wood	Lignum Guajaci (Guajakholz)
Gum Acacia	Acaciae Gummi (arabisches Gummi)
Hamamelis bark	Cortex Hamamelidis (Hamamelisrinde)
- leaves	Hamamelidis folia (Hamamelisblätter)
- ointment	Ungt. Hamamelidis (Hamamelissalbe)
Heavy Magnesia	Magnesia ponderosa (gebrannte Magnesia)
- Magnesium Carbonate	Magnesii Carbonas ponderosus (kohlensaure Magnesia)
Hemidesmus root	Hemidesmi radix (Hemidesmuswurzel)
Hemlock	Conii folia (Schierling)
Henbane leaves	Hyoscyami folia (Bilsenkraut)
Hepatic Aloes	Aloe socotrina (Sansibaraloe)
Hoffmann's Anodyne	Spiritus Aetheris comp. (zusammengesetzte Hoffmannstropfen)
Homatropine discs	Lamellae Homatropinae (Homatropinlamellen)
Hops	Lupulus (Hopfen)
Horseradish root	Armoraciae radix (Meerrettichwurzel)
Hydrastis rhizome	Hydrastis rhizoma (Gelbwurzel)
Hydrobromate of Homatropine	Homatropinae hydrobromidum (bromsaures Homatropin)

— 37 —

Hydrochlorate of Apomorphine	Apomorphinae hydrochloridum (salzsaures Apomorphin)
- - Morphine	Morphinae Hydrochloridum (salzsaures Morphium)
- - Quinine	Quininae Hydrochloridum (salzsaures Chinin)
Hydrochloric acid	Acid. hydrochloricum (Salzsäure)
Hydrogen Borate	Acid. boricum (Borsäure)
Hydrous wool fat	Adeps lanae hydrosus (Lanolin)
Hyoscine Hydrobromide	Hyoscinae Hydrobromidum (bromsaures Hyoscin)
Hyoscyamine Sulphate	Hyoscyaminae Sulphas (schwefelsaures Hyosciamin)
Hyoscyamus leaves	Folia Hyoscyami (Bilsenkraut)
Hypodermic injection	Injectio hypodermica (Einspritzung)
- - of Apomorphine	- - Apomorphinae (Apomorphineinspritzung)
- - - Cocaine	Injectio hypodermica Cocainae (Kokaineinspritzung)
- - - Ergot	Injectio hypodermica Ergotae (Mutterkornextrakteinspritzung)
- - - Morphine	Injectio hypodermica Morphinae (Morphiumeinspritzung)
India rubber	Caoutchouc (Kautschuk)
Indian Hemp	Cannabis indica (indischer Hanf)
Infusion of Bearberry	Infusum Uvae Ursi (Bärentraubenblätteraufguß)
Infusion of Broom	Infusum Scoparii (Ginsteraufguß)
- - Buchu	- Buchu (Buchublätteraufguß)
- - Calumba	- Calumbae (Colombowurzelaufguß)
- - Cascarilla	- Cascarillae (Cascarillarindenaufguß)
- - Chiretta	- Chiratae (Chirettakrautaufguß)
- - Cloves	- Caryophylli (Nelkenaufguß)
- - Cusparia	- Cuspariae (Cuspariarindenaufguß)

— 38 —

Infusion of Digitalis	Infusum Digitalis (Fingerhut=blätteraufguß)
- - Ergot	- Ergotae (Mutterkorn=aufguß)
- - Hops	- Lupuli (Hopfenauf=guß)
- - Krameria	- Krameriae (Ratan=hiawurzelaufguß)
- - Quassia	- Quassiae (Quassia=holzaufguß)
- - Rhubarb	- Rhei (Rhabarberauf=guß)
- - Senega	- Senegae(Senegawur=zelaufguß)
- - Senna	- Sennae (Sennesblät=teraufguß)
- - Serpentary	- Serpentariae(Schlan=genwurzelaufguß)
Jodine	Jodum (Jod)
- ointment	Ungt. Jodi (Jodsalbe)
Jodoform ointment	- Jodoformi (Jodoform=salbe)
- suppositories	Suppositoria Jodoformi (Jodo=form Suppositorien)
Ipecacuanha root	Radix Ipecacuanhae (Brech=wurzel)
- lozenge	Trochiscus Ipecacuanhae (Ipecacuanhapastille)
- - with Morphine	Trochiscus Morphinae et Ipecacuanhae (Morphiumipe=cacuanhapastille)
- wine	Vinum Ipecacuanhae (Brech=wein)
Iron	Ferrum (Eisen)
- and Ammonium Citrate	Ferri et Ammonii Citras (citro=nensaures Eisenammonium)
- - Quinine Citrate	Ferri et Quininae Citras (citro=nensaures Eisenchinin)
- Arsenate	- arsenas (arsensaures Eisen)
- Phosphate	- phosphas (phosphorsaures Eisen)
- pill	Pilula ferri (Blaudsche Pillen)
- - with Aloes	- aloes et ferri (Aloe=eisenpille)
- lozenge	Trochiscus ferri reducti (Eisen=pastille)

Iron Sulphate	Ferri sulphas (Eisenvitriol)
- wine	Vinum ferri (Eisenwein)
Jaborandi leaves	Jaborandi folia (Joborand=blätter)
Jalap	Jalapa (Jalapenknollen)
- resin	Jalapae resina (Jalapenharz)
Jiuce of Belladonna	Succus Belladonnae (frischer Tollkirschenkrautsaft)
- - Broom	- Scoparii (frischer Ginster=saft)
- - Conium	- Conii (frischer Schierlings=saft)
- - Hyoscyamus	- Hyoscyami (frischer Bilsenkrautsaft)
- - Lemon	- Limonis (frischer Citro=nensaft)
- - Taraxacum	- Taraxaci (Löwenzahnwur=zelsaft)
Juniper tar oil	Oleum cadinum (Wachholder=teeröl)
Kaolin	Kaolinum (gereinigtes Alumi=niumsilicat)
Krameria root	Krameriae radix (Ratanhia=wurzel)
- lozenge	Trochiscus Krameriae (Ra=tanhiapastille)
Lactic acid	Acidum lacticum (Milchsäure)
Lactose	Saccharum lactis (Milchzucker)
Lard	Adeps (Schmalz)
Lead acetate	Plumbi acetas (essigsaures Blei)
- - ointment	Ungt. plumbi acetatis (Blei=salbe)
- Carbonate	Plumbi Carbonas (kohlensau=res Blei)
- - ointment	Ungt. Plumbi carbonatis (koh=lensaure Bleisalbe)
- Jodide	Plumbi jodidum (Jodblei)
- - ointment	Ungt. plumbi jodidi (Jodblei=salbe)
- - plaster	Emplastrum Plumbi jodidi (Jodbleipflaster)
Lead Oxide	Plumbi oxidum (Silberglätte)
- Plaster	Emplastrum Plumbi (Blei=pflaster)
- subacetate ointment	Ungt. Glycerini plumbi subace-tatis (Bleisalbe mit Glycerin)

— 40 —

Leeches	Hirudines (Blutegel)
Lemon Jiuce	Succus Limonis (Citronenſaft)
- Peel	Limonis Cortex (Citronenſchale)
Light Calcined Magnesia	Magnesia levis (gebrannte Magneſia)
- Magnesia	Magnesia levis (gebrannte Magneſia)
- Magnesium Carbonate	Magnesii Carbonas levis (kohlenſaure Magneſia)
- - Oxide	Magnesia levis (gebrannte Magneſia)
Lime	Calx (Kalk)
- water	Liquor Calcis (Kalkwaſſer)
Liniment of Aconite	Linimentum Aconiti (Akonitliniment)
- - Ammonia	- Ammoniae (flüchtiges Liniment)
- - Belladonna	- Belladonnae (Belladonnaliniment)
- - Camphor	- Camphorae (Kampferöl)
- - Chloroform	- Chloroformi (Chloroformliniment)
- - Croton oil	- Crotonis (Krotonölliniment)
Liniment of Jodine	Liquor Jodi fortis (ſtarke Jodtinktur)
- - Lime	Linimentum Calcis (Kalkwaſſer u. Öl)
- - Mercury	- Hydrargyri (Queckſilberliniment)
- - Mustard	- Sinapis (Senfliniment)
- - Opium	- Opii (Opiumliniment)
- - Potassium Jodide with soap	- Potassi jodidi cum sapone (Jodkaliumſeifenliniment)
- - Turpentine	- Terebinthinae (Terpentinliniment)
- - - and acetic acid	- Terebinthinae aceticum (eſſigſaures Terpentinliniment)
Linseed	Semen Lini (Leinſamen)
- oil	Oleum Lini (Leinöl)
Liquefied Phenol	Acid. carbol. liquef. (flüſſige Karbolſäure)

— 41 —

Liquid Extract of Actaea racemosa	Extractum Cimicifugae liquidum (flüssiges Cimicifugenwurzelextrakt)
- - - Belladonna	Extr. Belladonnae liq. (flüssiges Belladonnaextrakt)
- - - Cascara sagrada	- Cascar. sagr. liq. (flüssiges Cascaraextrakt)
- - - Cimicifuga	- Cimicifugae liq. (flüssiges Cimicifugenwurzelextrakt)
- - - Cinchona	- Cinchonae liquid. (flüssiges Chinarindenextrakt)
- - - Coca	- Cocae liquid (flüssiges Kofusblätterextrakt)
- - - Ergot	- Ergotae liquid (flüssiges Mutterkornextrakt)
- - - Hamamelis	- Hamamelidis liquidum (flüssiges Hamamelisblätterextrakt)
- - - Hydrastis	- Hydrastis fluidum (flüssiges Hydrastiswurzelextrakt)
- - - Ipecacuanha	- Ipecacuanhae fluidum (flüssiges Brechwurzelextrakt)
- - - Jaborandi	- Jaborandi fluidum (flüssiges Jaborandenblätterextrakt)
- - - Liquorice	- Glyzyrrhizae fluidum (flüssiges Süßholzextrakt)
- - - Male fern	- Filicis fluidum (flüssiges Farnwurzelextrakt)
- - - Nux vomica	- Nucis vomicae fluidum (flüssiges Brechnußextrakt)
- - - Opium	- Opii fluidum (flüssiges Opiumextrakt)
- - - Pareira	- Pareirae fluidum (flüssiges Grieswurzelextrakt)
- - - Sarsaparilla	- Sarsaparillae fluidum (flüssiges Sarsaparillenwurzelextrakt)
- - - Taraxacum	- Taraxaci fluidum (flüssiges Löwenzahnwurzelextrakt)
- Glucose	Syrup Glucosi (Stärkesyrup)
Liquor Potassae arsenitis	Liquor arsenicalis (Fowlersche Tropfen)
Liquorice root	Glyzyrrhizae radix (Süßholzwurzel)
Litharge	Lithargyrum (Silberglätte)

Lithium Carbonate	Lithii Carbonas (kohlensaures Lithium)
- Citrate	- Citras (citronensaures Lithium)
Liver of Sulphur	Potassa sulphurata (Schwefelleber)
Logwood	Haematoxyli lignum (Blauholz)
Lunar caustic	Argenti Nitras (Silbernitrat)
Magnesium Carbonate	Magnesii Carbonas (kohlensaure Magnesia)
- Sulphate	- Sulphas (schwefelsaure Magnesia)
Male fern	Filix Mas (Farnwurzel)
Menthol plaster	Emplastrum Mentholi (Mentholpflaster)
Mercurial plaster	Emplastrum Hydrargyri (Quecksilberpflaster)
Mercuric Ammonium chloride	Hydrargyrum ammoniatum (weißer Präzipitat)
Mercuric chloride	Hydrargyri perchloridum (Sublimat)
- jodide	- jodidum rubrum (rotes Quecksilberjodid)
- - ointment	Ungt. Hydrargyri jod. rub. (rote Quecksilberjodidsalbe)
- nitrate ointment	- Hydrargyri nitratis (salpetersaure Quecksilbersalbe)
- oleate	Hydrargyri oleas (ölsaures Quecksilber)
- - ointment	Ungt. Hydrarg. oleatis (ölsaure Quecksilbersalbe)
Mercurous chloride	Hydrargyri subchloridum (Kalomel)
- - ointment	Ungt. Hydrargyri subchloridi (Kalomelsalbe)
Mercury	Hydrargyrum (Quecksilber)
- with Chalk	- c. Creta (Quecksilberkalkverreibung)
- ointment	Ungt. Hydrargyri (Quecksilbersalbe)
- pill	Pilula Hydrargyri (Quecksilberpille)
Mezereon bark	Mezerei cortex (Seidelbast)

Milk sugar	Saccharum Lactis (Milch=zucker)
- of Sulphur	Sulphur praecipitatum (Schwe=felmilch)
Mitigated caustic	Argenti nitras mitigatus (ver=dünnter Höllenstein)
Mixtur of Brandy	Mistura spiritus vini gallici (Cognacmixtur)
Morphine Lozenge	Trochiscus Morphinae (Mor=phiumpastille)
- - with Ipecacuanha	- Morphinae et Ipecacuanhae (Morphium= und Brechwurzelpastille)
- suppositories	Suppositoria Morphinae (Mor=phiumsuppositorien)
- Tartrate	Morphinae Tartras (weinsau=res Morphium)
Mucilage of Gum Acacia	Mucilago Acaciae (Gummi=schleim)
- - Tragacanth	- Tragacanthae (Tragant=schleim)
Musk	Moschus (Moschus)
Mustard	Semen Sinapis (Senf)
- poultice	Cataplasma Sinapis (Senfteig)
- paper	Charta sinapis (Senfpflaster)
Myrrh	Myrrha (Myrrhen)
Nitric acid	Acidum nitricum (Salpeter=säure)
Nitroglycerin tablets	Tabellae Trinitrini (Nitrogly=cerintabletten)
Nutmeg	Myristica (Muskatnuß)
Nux vomica	Nux vomica (Brechnuß)
Oil of Anise	Oleum Anisi (Anisöl)
- - Cade	- cadinum (Wachholder=teeröl)
- - Cajuput	- Cajeputi (Cajeputöl)
- - Caraway	- carvi (Kümmelöl)
- - Chamomile	- Chamomillae (Kamillenöl)
- - Cinnamom	- Cinnamomi (Zimtöl)
- - Cloves	- Caryophillorum (Nelkenöl)
- - Copaiba	- Copaibae (Kopaivaöl)
- - Coriander	- Coriandri (Korianderöl)
- - Cubebs	- Cubebae (Kubebenöl)
- - Dill	- Anethi (Dillöl)
- - Eucalyptus	- Eucalypti (Eucalyptusöl)
- - Juniper	- Juniperi (Wacholderöl)

— 44 —

Oil of Lavender	Oleum Lavendulae (Lavendelöl)
- - Lemon	- Limonis (Citronenöl)
- - Nutmeg	- Myristicae (Muskatnußöl)
- - Peppermint	- Menthae pip. (Pfeffer=minzöl)
- - Pimento	- Pimentae (Pimentöl)
- - Pine	- Pini (Latschenkieferöl)
- - Rose	- Rosae (Rosenöl)
- - Rosemary	- Rosmarini (Rosmarinöl)
- - Sandal wood - - Santal	- Santali (Sandelholzöl)
- - Spearmint	- Menthae viridis (grünes Pfefferminzöl)
- - Theobroma	- Theobromatis (Kakaoöl)
- - Turpentine	- Terebinthinae (Terpentinöl)
Oleic acid	Acid. oleicicum (Ölsäure)
Olive oil	Oleum Olivae (Olivenöl)
Opium plaster	Emplastrum Opii (Opium=pflaster)
Orange wine	Vinum Aurantii (Orangenwein)
- flower water	Aqua Amantii floris (Orangenblütenwasser)
Otte of Rose	Oleum Rosae (Rosenöl)
Oxymel of Squill	Oxymel Scillae (Meerzwiebel=honig)
Panama bark	Quillajae Cortex (Panama=späne)
Pancreatic solution	Liquor Pancreatis (Pancreas=lösung)
Para. acet. phenetidin.	Phenacetinum (Phenacetin)
Paregoric Elixir	Tinctura Camphorae comp. (zu=sammengesetzte Kampfertink=tur)
Pareira root	Pareirae radix (Grieswurzel)
Peppermint water	Aqua Menthae piperitae (Pfef=ferminzwasser)
Perchloride of mercury	Hydrargyrum perchloridum (Sublimat)
Phenol lozenge	Trochiscus acidi carbolici (Kar=bolsäurepastille)
- ointment	Ungt. ac. carbolici (Karbol=salbe)
- suppositories	Suppositoria acidi carbolici (Karbolsäuresuppositorien)
Phenyl of acetamide	Acetanilidum (Antifebrin)

Phosphorated oil	Oleum phosphoratum (Phosphoröl)
Phosphorous pill	Pilula phosphori (Phosphorpille)
Physostigminae Sulphate	Physostigminae Sulphas (schwefelsaures Eserin)
Pill of Aloes and Asafetida	Pilula Aloes et Asafetidae (Aloeasantpille)
- - Aloes and Iron	- Aloes et Ferri (Aloe- und Eisenpille)
- - - and Myrrh	- Aloes et Myrrhae (Aloe- und Myrrhenpille)
- - Barbados Aloes	- Aloes (Aloepille)
- - Colocynth and Hyoscyamus	- Colocynthidis et Hyoscyami (Koloquinten- und Bilsenkrautextraktpille)
- - Ipecacuanha with Squill	- Ipecacuanhae cum Scilla (Brechwurzel- und Meerzwiebelpille)
- - Lead with Opium	- Plumbi cum opio (Blei- und Opiumpille)
- - Quinine Sulphate	- Quininae sulphatis (Chininpille)
- - Socotrine Aloes	- Aloes socotrinae (Aloepille)
Pilocarpine Nitrate	Pilocarpinae Nitras (salpetersaures Pilocarpin)
Pimento	Pimenta (Piment)
- water	Aqua Pimentae (Pimentwasser)
Pitch plaster	Emplastrum Picis (Pechpflaster)
Plummer's pill	Pilula Hydrargyri subchloridi comp. (zusammengesetzte Kalomelpille)
Podophyllum rhizome ⎫ - root ⎭	Podophylli rhizoma (Podophyllwurzel)
- resin	- resina (Podophyllharz)
Pomegranate bark	Granati cortex (Granatwurzelrinde)
Poppy capsules	Papaveris capsulae (Mohnköpfe)
Potassium Acetate	Potassii Acetas (essigsaures Kali)
- Bicarbonate	- Bicarbonas (doppeltkohlensaures Kali)

Potassium Bromide	Potassii Bromidum (Bromkali)
- Carbonate	- Carbonas (kohlensaures Kali)
- Chlorate	- Chloras (chlorsaures Kali)
- - lozenge	Trochiscus potassii chloratis (Kalichloricumtablette)
- Citrate	Potassii Citras (citronensaures Kali)
- Hydrate	Potassa caustica (Ätzkali)
- Hydrogen Carbonate	Potassii bicarbonas (doppelkohlensaures Kali)
- Hydroxide	Potassa caustica (Ätzkali)
- Jodide	Potassium Jodidi (Jodkalium)
- - ointment	Ungt. Potassii jodidi (Jodkalisalbe)
- Nitrate	Potassii nitras (Salpeter)
- Permanganate	- permanganas (übermangansaures Kali)
- Sulphate	- sulphas (schwefelsaures Kali)
- Tartrate	- Tartras (weinsaures Kali)
Precipitated Calcium Carbonate - Chalk	Calcii Carbonas praecipitatus (kohlensaurer Kalk)
- Sulphur	Sulphur praecipitatum (Schwefelmilch)
Prepared chalk	Creta praeparata (präparierter Kalk)
- Coal tar	Pix Carbonis praeparata (gereinigter Kohlenteer)
- Storax	Styrax praeparatus (gereinigter Styrax)
- Suet	Sevum praeparatum (gereinigter Talg)
Prunes	Prunum (Pflaume)
Purified Cream of Tartar	Potassii tartras acidus (Kremortartari)
- Ether	Aether purificatus (gereinigter Äther)
- ox bile	Fel bovinum purificatum (gereinigte Ochsengalle)
Pyrethrum root	Pyrethri radix (Bertramswurzel)

Quassia wood	Quassiae lignum (Quassiaholz)
Quillaja bark	Quillajae cortex (Quillajarinde)
Quinine Hydrochloride	Quininae Hydrochloricum (salzsaures Chinin)
- Sulphate	Quininae Sulphas (schwefelsaures Chinin)
- Wine	Vinum Quininae (Chinawein)
Rectified Spirit	Spiritus rectificatus (90 % iger Alkohol)
Red Cinchona bark	Cinchonae rubrae cortex (Chinarinde)
- Mercuric Oxide	Hydrargyri oxidum rubrum (rotes Quecksilberoxyd)
- - - ointment	Ungt. Hydrargyri oxidi rubri (rote Quecksilberoxydsalbe)
- Poppy Petals	Rosae Gallicae petala (Rosenblätter)
- Sandal wood } - Sanders }	Pterocarpi lignum (rotes Sandelholz)
Reduced Iron	Ferrum redactum (reduziertes Eisen)
- - lozenge	Trochiscus ferri redacti (reduzierte Eisenpastille)
Refined Sugar	Saccharum purificatum (reiner Zucker)
Resin	Resina (dicker Terpentin)
- ointment	Ungt. Resinae (Terpentinsalbe)
- plaster	Emplastrum resinae (Heftpflaster)
Rhatany root	Krameriae radix (Ratanhiawurzel)
Rhubarb -	Rhei radix (Rhabarberwurzel)
Rochelle salt	Soda tartarata (Kaliumnatrontartrat)
Rose water	Aqua Rosae (Rosenwasser)
- - ointment	Ungt. aquae Rosae (Rosensalbe)
Saccharated Iron Carbonate	Ferri Carbonas saccharatus (Eisenzucker)
- solution of Lime	Liquor Calcis saccharatus (gezuckertes Kalkwasser)
Sacred bark	Cortex Cascara sagrada (Kaskararinde)

Saffron	Crocus (Safran)
Salicylic acid	Acid. salicylicum (Salicyl-säure)
- ointment	Ungt. ac. salicylici (Salicyl-salbe)
Salt of Tartrar	Potassii Carbonas (kohlensaures Kali)
Santonin lozenge	Trochiscus Santonini (Wurm-zeltchen)
Sassafras root	Sassafras radix (Sassafras-wurzel)
Scammony root	Scammoniae radix (Skammo-niawurzel)
Scopolamine Hydrobromide	Hyoscynae Hydrobromidum (bromsaures Hyoscin)
Seidlitz powder	Pulvis Sodae Tartarae effer-vescens (Seidlitzpulver)
Senega root	Senegae radix (Senegawurzel)
Serpentary rhizome	Serpentariae rhizoma (Schlangenwurzel)
Silver Nitrate	Argenti nitras (Höllenstein)
Slaked lime	Calcii Hydras (gelöschter Kalk)
Soap plaster	Emplastrum saponis (Seifen-pflaster)
Sodium Arsenate	Sodii Arsenas (arsensaures Natron)
- Benzoate	- Benzoas (benzoesaures Natron)
- Bicarbonate	- Bicarbonas (doppel-kohlensaures Natron)
- - lozenge	Trochiscus sodii bicarbonatis (doppelkohlensaure Natron-pastille)
- Bromide	Sodii Bromidum (bromsaures Natron)
- Carbonate	- Carbonas (kohlensaures Natron)
- Chloride	- Chloridum (Salz)
- Hypophosphite	- Hypophosphis (unter-phosphorsaures Natron)
- Jodide	- Jodidum (Jodnatrium)
- Nitrite	- Nitris (salpetersaures Natron)
- Phosphate	- Phosphas (phosphor-saures Natron)

— 49 —

Sodium Salicylate	Sodii Salicylas (falicylfaures Natron)
- Sulphate	- Sulphas (ſchwefelſaures Natron)
- Sulphite	- Sulphis (ſchwefligſaures Natron)
- Sulphocarbolate	- Sulpho carbolas (ſchwefelkarbolſaures Natron)
Solution of Ammonia	Liquor Ammoniae (Salmiak= geiſt)
- - Ammonium Acetate	Liq. Ammonii acetatis (eſſig= ſaure Ammoniumlöſung)
- - Arsenious and Mercury Jodide	Liquor Arsenii et Hydrargyri jodidi (Arſenjodquecksilber= löſung)
- - Atropine sulphate	Liquor Atropinae sulphatis (ſchwefelſaure Atropinlöſung)
- - Bismuth and Ammonium Citrate	Liquor Bismuthi et Ammonii citrici (citronenſaure Ammo= niak=Wismutlöſung)
- of chlorinated Soda	Liquor sodae chlorinatae (chlor= ſaure Natronlöſung)
- - Coal tar	Liquor picis carbonis (alko= holiſche Teerlöſung)
- - Ferric acetate	Liquor ferri acetatis (eſſigſaure Eiſenlöſung)
- - - chloride	- - perchloridi (Eiſen= chloridlöſung)
- - - nitrate	- - nitratis (ſalpeter= ſaure Eiſenlöſung)
- - - sulphate	Liquor ferri persulphatis (ſchwefelſaure Eiſenlöſung)
- - Hamamelis	Liquor Hamamelidis (alko= holiſcher Hamamelisblätter= auszug)
- - Hydrochlorate of Morphine	Liquor Morphinae hydro- chloridi (ſalzſaure Mor= phiumlöſung)
- - Hydrogen peroxide	Liquor hydrogenii peroxidi (Wasserſtoffſuperoxydlöſung)
- - India rubber	Liquor Caoutchouc (Gummi= löſung)
- - Lime	Liquor Calcis (Kalkwaſſer)
- - Magnesium Carbonate	Liquor Magnesii carbonatis (flüſſige kohlenſaure Magneſia)

Solution of Mercuric chloride	Liquor Hydrargyri perchloridi (Sublimatlösung)
- - Morphine Acetate	Liquor Morphinae acetatis (essigsaure Morphiumlösung)
- - - hydrochloride	Liquor Morphinae hydrochloridi (salzsaure Morphiumlösung)
- - - tartrate	Liquor Morphinae tartratis (weinsaure Morphiumlösung)
- - Nitroglycerin	Liquor trinitrini (Nitroglyzerinlösung)
- - Potash	- Potassae (Kalilaugelösung)
- - Potassium permanganate	- potassii permanganatis (übermangansaure Kalilösung)
- - Strychnine hydrochloride	Liquor Strychninae hydrochloridi (salzsaure Strychninlösung)
Spearmint water	Aqua Menthae viridis (grünes Pfefferminzwasser)
Spermaceti	Cetaceum (Wallrat)
- ointment	Ungt. Cetacei (Wallratsalbe)
Spirit of Anise	Spiritus Anisi (Anistropfen)
- - Cajuput	- Cajuputi (Cajeputtropfen)
- - Camphor	- Camphorae (Kampferspiritus)
- - Chloroform	- Chloroformi (Chloroformspiritus)
- - Cinnamom	- Cinnamomi (Zimttropfen)
- - Ether	- Aetheris (Hoffmanns tropfen)
- - Juniper	- Juniperi (Wachholderspiritus)
- - Lavender	- Lavandulae (Lavendelspiritus)
- - Nitrous Ether	- Aetheris nitrosi (versüßter Salpetergeist)
- - Nutmeg	- Myristicae (Muskatnußspiritus)
- - Peppermint	- Menthae piperitae (Pfefferminztropfen)
- - Rosemary	- Rosmarini (Rosmarintropfen)

— 51 —

Spirit of sal volatile	Spiritus Ammoniae aromatic. (aromatischer Salmiakgeist)
Squill	Scilla (Meerzwiebel)
Starch	Amylum (Stärke)
Stavesacre seeds	Staphisagriae semina (Stephanskörner)
- ointment	Ungt. Staphisagriae (Stephansalbe)
Stramonium leaves	Stramonii folia (Stechapfelblätter)
- seeds	- semina (Stechapfelsamen)
Strong solution of Ammonia	Liquor Ammoniae fortis (Salmiakgeist)
- - - Ferric chloride	- ferri perchloridi fortis (starke Eisenchloridlösung)
- - - Jodine	Liquor Jodi fortis (starke Jodtinktur)
- - - Lead subacetate	- Plumbi subacet. fortis (Bleiextrakt)
Strophantus seeds	Strophanti semina (Strophantussamen)
Strychnine	Strychnina (Strychnin)
- Hydrochloride	Strychninae Hydrochloridum (salzsaures Strychnin)
Subchloride of Mercury	Hydrargyri subchloridum (Kalomel)
Sublimed Sulphur	Sulphur sublimatum (Schwefelblüte)
Sucrose	Saccharum purificatum (reiner Zucker)
Sulphur Jodide	Sulphuris Jodidum (Jodschwefel)
- - ointment	Ungt. sulphuris jodidi (Jodschwefelsalbe)
- Lozenge	Trochiscus Sulphuris (Schwefelpastille)
- ointment	Ungt. Sulphuris (Schwefelsalbe)
Sulphurated Antimony	Antimonium sulphuratum (Goldschwefel)
- Potash	Potassa sulphurata (Schwefelleber)
Sulphuric acid	Acidum sulphuricum (Schwefelsäure)

4*

— 52 —

Sulphurous acid	Acidum sulphurosum (ſchweflige Säure)
Sumbul root	Sumbul radix (Moſchuswurzel)
Sweet Almond	Amygdala dulcis (ſüße Mandel)
- spirit of Nitre	Spiritus Aetheris nitrosi (verſüßter Salpetergeiſt)
Syrup of balsam of Tolu	Syrupus tolutanus (Tolubalſamſirup)
- - Calcium Lactophosphate	- Calcii lactophosphatis (milchphosphorſaurer Kalkſirup)
- - Chloral	Syrup. Chloral (Chloralhydratſirup)
- - Codeine	- Codeinae (Kodeinſirup)
- - Ferrous Jodide	- ferri jodidi (Jodeiſenſirup)
- - - Phosphate	- ferri phosphati (phosphorſaurer Eiſenſirup)
- - Ginger	- Zingiberis (Ingwerſirup)
- - Glucose	- Glucosi (Stärkeſirup)
- - Hemidesmus	- Hemidesmi (Hemidesmuswurzelſirup)
- - Lemon	- Limonis (Citronenſirup)
- - Orange flower	- Aurantii floris (Orangenblütenſirup)
- - Phosphate of Iron with Quinine and Strychnine	- Ferri phosphatis cum Quinina et Strychnina (phosphorſaurer Eiſenſirup mit Chinin und Strychnin)
- of Red Poppy	- Rhoeados (Klatſchroſenſirup)
- - Rhubarb	- Rhei (Rhabarberſirup)
- - Roses	- Rosae (Roſenſirup)
- - Senna	- Sennae (Sennesblätterſirup)
- - Squill	- Scillae (Meerzwiebelſirup)
- - Virginian prune	- Pruni virginianae (virginiſcher Pflaumenbaumrindenſirup)
Tablets of Nitroglycerin	Tabellae Trinitrini (Nitroglyzerintabletten)
Tamarinds	Tamarindus (Tamarinden)

— 53 —

Tannic acid	Acidum tannicum (Gerbſäure)
- - lozenge	Trochiscus acidi tannici (Gerb=ſäurepaſtille)
- - suppositories	Suppositoria acidi tannici (Gerbſäureſuppoſitorien)
Tar.	Pix liquida (flüſſiges Pech)
- ointment	Ungt. picis liquid. (Teerſalbe)
Taraxacum root	Taraxaci radix (Löwenzahn=wurzel)
Tartarated Antimony	Antimonium tartaratum (Brechweinſtein)
- Iron	Ferrum tartaratum (weinſaures Eiſen)
- Soda	Soda tartarata (weinſaures Natron)
Tartaric acid	Acidum tartaricum (Weinſtein=ſäure)
Tartrate of Potassium and Sodium	Soda tartarata (Kalium=natriumtartrat)
Terebene	Terebenum (Tereben)
Theine	Caffeina (Koffein)
Thus americanum	Frankincense (Harz von pinus palustris)
Tincture of Aconite	Tinctura Aconiti (Akonit=tinktur)
- - Actaea racemosa	- Cimicifugae (Cimi=cifugatinktur)
- - Aloes	- Aloes (Aloetinktur)
- - Arnica	- Arnicae (Arnika=tinktur)
- - Asafetida	- Asafetidae (Stinka=ſanttinktur)
- - Balsam of Tolu	- tolutana (Tolubal=ſamtinktur)
- - Belladonna	- Belladonnae (Toll=kirſchenblättertinktur)
- - Buchu	- Buchu (Buchublätter=tinktur)
- - Calumba	- Calumbae (Kolombo=wurzeltinktur)
- - Cantharides	- Cantharidis (Kan=tharidentinktur)
- - Capsicum	- Capsici (ſpaniſch=Pfeffertinktur)
- - Cascarilla	- Cascarillae (Kas=karillrindentinktur)

Tincture of Catechu	Tinctura Catechu (Katechu=tinktur)
- - Chiretta	- Chiratae (Chiratta=tinktur)
- - Cimicifuga	- Cimicifugae (Cimi=cifugatinktur)
- - Cinchona	- Cinchonae (China=rindentinktur)
- - Cinnamom	- Cinnamomi (Zimt=tinktur)
- - Cochineal	- Cocci (Kochenille=tinktur)
- - Colchicum seeds	- Colchici seminum (Kolchikumtinktur)
- - Conium	- Conii (Schierlings=[Frucht=]tinktur)
- - Cubebs	- Cubebae (Kubeben=tinktur)
- - Digitalis	- Digitalis (Fingerhut=tinktur)
- - Ferric chloride	- Ferri per chloridi (Eisen=chloridtinktur)
- - Gelsemium	- Gelsemii (Gelsemium=wurzeltinktur)
- - Ginger	- Zingiberis (Ingwertink=tur)
- - Hamamelis	- Hamamelidis (Hama=melistinktur)
- - Hops	- Lupuli (Hopfentinktur)
- - Hydrastis	- Hydrastis (Hydrastis=tinktur)
- - Hyoscyamus	- Hyoscyami (Bilsen=krauttinktur)
- - Indian Hemp	- Cannabis indicae (in=dische Hanftinktur)
- - Jaborandi	- Jaborandi (Jaboran=denblättertinktur)
- - Jalap	- Jalapae (Jalapentink=tur)
- - Jodine	- Jodi (Jodtinktur)
- - Kino	- Kino (Kinotinktur)
- - Krameria	- Krameriae (Ratanha=wurzeltinktur)
- - Lemon	- Limonis (Citronentink=tur)

Tincture of Myrrh	Tinctura Myrrhae (Myrrhen= tinktur)
- - Nux vomica	- nucis vomicae (Brech= nußtinktur)
- - Opium	- Opii (Opiumtinktur)
- - Orange	- Aurantii (Orangentink= tur)
- - Podophyllum	- Podophylli (Podophyl= lumharztinktur)
- - Pyrethrum	- Pyrethri (Bertrams= wurzeltinktur)
- - Quassia	- Quassiae (Quassiaholz= tinktur)
- - Quillaia	- Quillaiae (Quillajarin= dentinktur)
- - Quinine	- Quininae (salzsaureChi= nintinktur)
- - Senega	- Senegae (Senegawur= zeltinktur)
- - Serpentary	- Serpentariae (Schlan= genwurzeltinktur)
- - Squill	- Scillae (Meerzwiebel= tinktur)
- - Stramonium	- Stramonii (Stechapfel= blättertinktur)
- - Strophantus	- Strophanti (Strophan= tussamentinktur)
- - Sumbul	- Sumbul (Moschuswur= zeltinktur)
- - Tolu	- tolutana (Tolubalsam= tinktur)
- - Virginian prune	- pruni Virginianae (vir= ginische Pflaumen= rindentinktur)
Toughened Caustic	Argenti Nitras induratus (Höl= lenstein mit Salpeter)
Tragacanth	Tragacantha (Tragant)
Trinitrin tablets	Tabellae Trinitrini (Nitrogly= cerintabletten)
Valerian rhizome	Valerianae rhizoma (Baldrian= wurzel)
Veratrine	Veratrina (Veratrin)
- ointment	Ungt. Veratrinae (Veratrin= salbe)

Vinegar of Cantharides	Acetum Cantharidis (Spanischer Fliegenessig)
- - Ipecacuanha	- Ipecacuanhae (Brechwurzelessig)
- - Squill	- Scillae (Meerzwiebelessig)
Volatile oil of Mustard	Oleum Sinapis aeth. (ätherisches Senföl)
Warming plaster	Emplastrum calefaciens (Rheumatismuspflaster)
White arsenic	Acidum arsenicosum (arsenige Säure)
- beeswax	Cera alba (weißes Wachs)
- mustard seed	Sinapis albae semina (weißer Senf)
- Precipitate	Hydrargyrum ammoniatum (weißes Quecksilberpräcipitat)
- - ointment	Ungt. Hydrargyri ammoniati (weiße Quecksilbersalbe)
Witch Hazel bark	Hamamelidis Cortex (Hamamelisrinde)
- - leaves	- Folia (Hamamelisblätter)
Wood charcoal	Carbo ligni (Lindenkohle)
Wool fat	Adeps lanae (Lanolin)
Yellow bees wax	Cera flava (gelbes Wachs)
- mercurial lotion	Lotio Hydrargyri flava (gelbes Quecksilberwaschwasser)
- mercuric oxide ointment	Ungt. Hydrargyri oxidi flavi (gelbe Quecksilbersalbe)
- wash	Lotio hydrargyri flava (gelbes Quecksilberwaschwasser)
Zanzibar Aloes	Socotrine Aloes (Sansibaraloe)
Zinc Acetate	Zinci Acetas (essigsaures Zink)
- Carbonate	- Carbonas (kohlensaures Zink)
- Chloride	- Chloridum (Chlorzink)
- oleate ointment	Ungt. Zinci oleatis (ölsaure Zinksalbe)
- ointment	Ungt. Zinci (Zinksalbe)
- oxide	Zinci oxidum (Zinkoxyd)
- sulphate	Zinci sulphas (schwefelsaures Zink)

Zinc sulphocarbolate	Zinci sulphocarbolas (schwefel= karbolsaures Zink)
- valerianate	- valerianas (baldriansau= res Zink)

VIII.
Das englische Rezept.
1. Beispiele aus der englischen Rezeptur.

Rp. Sodium bromide ℥ ss
Ammoniated Tincture of Valerian ʒ I
Syrup of Orange ʒ I
Distilled water ad ℥ VIII

Tincture of Rhubarb. ʒ I
Compound tincture of Cinchona ʒ I
Liquid Extract of Condurango ʒ III

Boric acid ʒ I
Hydrous wool fat
Soft Paraffin ān. ℥ ss
Oil of Lavender m. VIII

Potassium chlorate ℥ ss
Compound tincture of Cardamom ʒ II
Distilled water ad ℥ X

Zinc sulphate gr. I
Distilled water ʒ III

Boric acid ℥ I
Distilled water ℥ X

Zinc sulphocarbolate ʒ ss
Distilled water ℥ VII

Alcoholic extract of Belladonna gr. I
Oil of Theobroma ʒ ss

Oil of Juniper ʒ II
Strong solution of Ammonia ℥ I
Olive oil ℥ IV

Quinine sulphate gr. VI
Reduced Iron gr. VI
Liquorice root
- extract aā. gr. ss
Extract of Taraxacum q. s.

Carbonate of Magnesium
Senna leaves.
Cream of Tartar.
Sugar aā. ℥ ss.

2. Die englische Signatur.

a) Allgemeine Ausdrücke.

nach Anweisung	as directed
wie bisher	as before
zum inneren Gebrauch	for internal use
einzunehmen	to be taken
einen Dessertlöffel voll	a dessertspoonful
- Eßlöffel voll	a tablespoonful
- Teelöffel voll	a teaspoonful
einige Tropfen	few drops
zehn bis zwanzig Tropfen	ten to twenty drops
den dritten, achten 2c. Teil	the third, eighth part
bei Bedürfnis	when required
gelegentlich	occasionally
täglich	daily
morgens	in the morning
abends	at bedtime
vor, nach dem Essen	before, after meals
ein-, zwei-, dreimal	once, twice, three times
zum äußerlichen Gebrauch	for external use
nur zum äußerlichen Gebrauch	- - - only
Vorsicht!	caution!
Gift!	poison!
umschütteln!	shake, to be shaken
verdünnen!	to be diluted!

b) Beispiele englischer Signaturen.

dreimal täglich 20 Tropfen vor dem Essen zu nehmen	twenty drops to be taken three times daily before meals
abends einen Eßlöffel voll zu nehmen zum Schlafen	a tablespoonful to be taken at bedtime for making sleep

alle vier Stunden den achten Teil zu nehmen — the eighth part to be taken every four hours
die Salbe ist jeden zweiten Abend einzureiben — use the ointment every second night
täglich mehrmals damit zu gurgeln — to be used as a gargle several times daily
zum Einreiben der schmerzenden Teile — to be rubbed on the painful spot
im Bedürfnis 20 Tropfen zu nehmen — take twenty drops when required
gelegentlich als leichtes Abführmittel zu gebrauchen — to be taken occasionally as a light aperient

c) Abkürzungen auf englischen Rezepten.

Abs. feb.	absente febre	wenn fieberfrei
Ad 2 vic.	ad duas vices	auf zweimal zu nehmen
Ad def. animi	ad defectionem animi	bis Ohnmacht
Ad del animi	ad deliquium animi	
Adst. febr.	adstante febre	während des Fiebers
Ad 3 tiam vic.	ad tertiam vicem	für dreimal
Aggred. febre	aggrediente febre	während des Eintritts des Fiebers
Alt. hor.	alternis horis	zweistündlich
Alvo adst.	alvo adstricta	bei Verstopfung
A. J.	ante jentaculum	nüchtern
A. P.	ante prandium	vor der Mahlzeit
B. M.	balneum mare	ein See- oder Salzbad
B. P.	British Pharmacopœia	nach dem englischen Arzneibuch
B. T.	balneum tepidum	ein warmes Bad
B. V.	balneum vaporis	ein Dampfbad
Cap.	capiat	lasse den Kranken einnehmen
Coch.	cochleare	ein Löffel voll
Coch. ampl.	„ amplum	ein Eßlöffel voll
„ mag.	„ magnum	
„ inf.	„ infantis	ein Kaffeelöffel voll
Cochleat.	cochleatim	löffelweise
C. v.	cras vespere	morgen Abend
C. m. s.	cras mane sumendu	morgen früh einzunehmen
De d. in d.	de die in diem	von Tag zu Tag
Dieb. alt.	diebus alternis	jeden zweiten Tag

Dieb. tert.	diebus tertiis	jeden dritten Tag
Diluc.	diluculo	bei Tagesanbruch
Donec alv. bis dej.	donec alvus bis dejiciatur	bis nach der zweiten Ausleerung
Donec alv. sol. fuer.	donec alvus soluta fuerit	bis Öffnung erfolgt
Febr. dur.	febre durante	während des Fiebers
Fem. intern.	femoribus internis	auf der inneren Seite der Schenkel
H. d.	horæ decubitus	beim Schlafengehen
Hor. interm.	horis intermediis	in den Zwischenstunden
H. s.	hora somni	gerade vor dem Schla=
H. s. s.	hora somni sumendu	fengehen zu nehmen
Hor. un. spat.	horae unius spatio	nach Verlauf einer Stunde
Hor. 11ma mat.	hora undecima matutina	elf Uhr früh
Ind.	indies	täglich
Inj. enem.	injiciatur enema	ein Klistier geben
Lat. dol.	lateri dolenti	auf die schmerzliche Seite
Man.	manipulus	eine Hand voll
Mane pr.	mane primo	morgens früh
Mod. præs.	modo præscripto	nach Vorschrift
Mor. dict.	more dicto	
Mor. sol.	more solito	wie gewöhnlich
Omn. hor.	omni hora	stündlich
Omn. bid.	omni biduo	alle zwei Tage
Omn. bih.	omni bihorio	alle zwei Stunden
O. m.	omni mane	jeden Morgen zu
O. m. s.	omni mane sumendu	nehmen
O. n.	omni nocte	jede Nacht
Omn. quad. hor.	omni quadrante hora	jede Viertelstunde
Part. aff.	partem affectam	der angegriffene Teil
Part. dolen.	partem dolentem	wo der Schmerz ist
P. rat. æt.	pro ratione ætatis	je nach dem Alter
P. r. n.	pro re nata	nach Umständen
Part. vic.	partibus vicibus	in geteilten Dosen
Q. l.	quantum libet	so viel wie beliebt
Q. p.	„ placet	

Q. q. h.	quaque quatuor horæ	alle vier Stunden
Q. s.	quantum satis seu sufficiat	so viel wie nötig
Repet.	repetatur	wiederholen
S. n. val.	si non valeat	bei Nichterfolg
Si op. sit.	si opus sit	wenn nötig ist
Si vir. perm.	si vires permittant	wenn es die Kräfte zu=lassen
Usq. ut. lig. anim.	usque ut liguerit animus	bis Ohnmacht
vom. urg.	vomitone urgente	wenn das Erbrechen lästig wird

IX.

Englische Gewichte, Hohl= und Längenmaße und ihre Beziehung zu den deutschen.

a grain	gr.	
a scruple	Ɔ	= 20 gr.
a drachm	ʒ	= Ɔ III
an ounce	℥	= ʒ VIII
a minim	m	
a fluid drachm	fl. ʒ	= 60 m.
a fluid ounce	fl. ℥	= fl. ʒ VIII
a pint	O	= fl. ℥ XX
half a scruple	Ɔ ss	
half a drachm	ʒ ss	
half an ounce	℥ ss	

Es sollen alle Flüssigkeiten gewogen werden. Trotzdem werden sie in der Regel von dem englischen Rezeptar gemessen, obwohl er dies eigentlich nur dann tun darf, wenn ℥ auf dem Rezept vermerkt ist.

Gewichte.

1 grain	gr.	
1 ounce	oz.	= 437.5 grains
1 pound	lb.	= 7000 "

Hohlmaße.

1 minim . . . . . m.
1 fluid drachm . . fl. drm. = 60 minims
1 fluid ounce . . fl. oz. = 8 fluid drachms
1 pint. . . . . . O. = 20 fluid ounces
1 gallon . . . . C. = 8 pints

Die ounce (Unze) der British Pharmacopœia unterscheidet sich von der ounce des Apothecary's or Troy weight, insofern die erstere 437.5 grains, die letztere 480 grains enthält. Die Gewichte der B. P. sind eben avoirdupois weight.

1 pound = 453.5925 Gramm
1 ounce = 28.3495 „
1 grain = 0.0648 „

1 Milligramm = 0.015432 grains
1 Centigramm = 0.15432 „
1 Decigramm = 1.5432 „
1 Gramm = 15.432 „
1 Kilogramm = 15432.348 „
 1 Ko. = 2 pds. 3 oz. 119.8 gr.

1 gallon = 4.543487 Liter
1 pint = 0.567936 „
1 fluid ounce = 0.028396 „
1 fluid drachm = 0.003549 „
1 minim = 0.000059 „

Längenmaße.

1 Inch = in
1 Foot = ft = 12 inches
1 Yard = yd = 36 inches

1 Inch = 0,025 m
1 Foot = 0,304 m
1 Yard = 0,914 m

X.
Münzsorten.

1. Half a penny	= $1/24$ s =	5 Pfennige.		
2. a penny	= $1/12$ s =	10	-	
3. two pences	= $1/6$ s =	20	-	
4. six pences	= $1/2$ s =	50	-	
5. one shilling	= 1 s =	1 Mark		
6. two shillings	= 2 s =	2	-	
7. half a crown	= $2^{1}/_{2}$ s =	2	-	50 Pfg.
8. ten shillings	= 10 s =	10	-	
9. a sovereign	= 20 s =	20	-	
10. a guinea	= 21 s =	21	-	
11. one pound	= 20 s =	20	-	
12. a five pound's note	= 100 s =	100	-	

1. und 2. sind Kupfermünzen,
4., 5., 6. und 7. sind Silbermünzen,
8., 9., 10. und 11. sind Goldmünzen,
12. ist Papiergeld.

Die beigesetzten Werte in deutschem Gelde entsprechen nicht dem Kurs, sondern ziehen nur einen Vergleich mit den bei uns üblichen Münzsorten.

XI.
Gespräche.

Good morning, Sir!	Guten Morgen, mein Herr!
Good morning.	Guten Morgen.
Please make me up this prescription.	Machen Sie mir bitte dies Rezept.
Very well.	Sehr wohl.

Can you make me up this prescription?	Können Sie mir dies Rezept wohl machen?
Yes, Sir, with pleasure.	Jawohl, sehr gern.
What time will it be ready?	Wann wird es fertig sein?
In about half an hour.	In einem halben Stündchen.
Than I call in again.	Dann komme ich wieder.

Will you be kind enough to send me this ointment?	Wollen Sie mir wohl diese Salbe senden?
Yes, Sir, where shall I send it to?	Ja, mein Herr, wo darf ich sie hinsenden?
My office is C....street No. 2 second floor.	Mein Comptoir ist C... straße Nr. 2, zweite Etage.

What's your best german preparation for corns?	Was ist das beste deutsche Präparat für Hühneraugen?
Well, do you want a liquid or a plaster?	Ja, wollen Sie eine Flüssigkeit oder ein Pflaster?
What is the most convenient?	Was ist am bequemsten?
I would prefer the plaster.	Ich würde das Pflaster vorziehen.
Then let me have a small box of the plaster.	Dann geben Sie mir eine kleine Schachtel von dem Pflaster.

Do you keep mineral waters?	Führen Sie Mineralwasser?
Yes, Sir, what water do you like to have?	Jawohl, mein Herr, welches Wasser wünschen Sie?
Apenta, you know, the well recommended aperient water.	Apenta, das viel empfohlene abführende Wasser, Sie wissen.
Very well, Sir, I have it in stock.	Jawohl, mein Herr, ich habe es vorrätig.
Then I want two large bottles.	Dann wünsche ich zwei große Flaschen.

What is the best thing for cough?	Was ist am besten gegen Husten?
Well, what do you like the best? Lozenges, drops, a mixture...?	Ja, was mögen Sie am liebsten? Pastillen, Tropfen, eine Mixtur...?
Anything, only it must be really efficacious.	Irgend etwas, wenn es nur hilft.
Then I recommend you these pastilles.	Dann empfehle ich Ihnen diese Pastillen.
How are they to be taken?	Wie sind dieselben zu nehmen?
One lozenge every two hours.	Zweistündlich eine Pastille.
They don't taste badly, I suppose?	Sie schmecken doch nicht schlecht?
Not at all.	Durchaus nicht.

My stomach is wrong, can you give me anything, to make me all right.	Ich habe mir den Magen verdorben; können Sie mir etwas geben, um mich wieder auf den Posten zu bringen?
Yes, Sir, try this powder.	Jawohl, versuchen Sie mal dies Pulver?
How is it to be taken?	Wie ist es zunehmen?
Three times daily.	Dreimal täglich.
Before or after meals?	Vor oder nach dem Essen?
Half an hour after meals.	Eine halbe Stunde nach dem Essen.
With or without water?	Mit oder ohne Wasser?
In half a tumbler full of water.	In einem halben Glase Wasser.

How do you sell Beecham's pills in Germany?	Wie verkaufen Sie in Deutschland Beecham's pills?
1,50 Mk. the small, 2,75 Mk. the large size.	1,50 Mk. die kleinen, 2,75 Mk. die größeren Schachteln.
That's a great difference between England and here.	Das ist ein großer Unterschied zwischen England und hier.
Well, you must consider duty, postage...	Ja, Sie müssen bedenken Zoll, Fracht...
Yes, certainly, never mind, let me have the 2,75 Mk. size.	Ja, natürlich, selbstverständlich, geben Sie mir eine 2,75 Mk.-Schachtel.

I have a beastly headache, have you anything against the pain?	Ich habe schauderhafte Kopfschmerzen, haben Sie nicht etwas dagegen?
Yes, Sir, I give you two powders, the one is to be taken at once, the other in the course of the day.	Jawohl, mein Herr, hier sind zwei Pulver, das eine nehmen Sie gleich, das andere im Laufe des Tages.
Thank you, good bye!	Danke sehr, adieu!
Good bye, Sir!	Adieu!

What do you think the best thing for toothache?	Was halten Sie für am besten gegen Zahnschmerzen?
Well, have you a hollow tooth or are you suffering from neuralgic pain?	Ja, haben Sie einen hohlen Zahn oder leiden Sie an neuralgischen Schmerzen?
No, only this very tooth is hollow.	Nein, nur gerade dieser Zahn ist hohl.
Then try this toothache-wadding.	Dann nehmen Sie diese Zahnwatte.

Will that help me?	Wird das helfen?
Yes, Sir, this wading is a realy good thing for toothache.	Jawohl, diese Watte ist wirklich gut gegen Zahnschmerzen.

I have caught a very bad cold.	Ich habe mich tüchtig erkältet.
Sorry to hear it.	Bedaure sehr.
What shall I do?	Was macht man dagegen?
Take a good strong dose of Aspirin.	Nehmen Sie eine ordentliche Dosis Aspirin.
What's that?	Was ist das?
A powder, to be taken with water.	Ein Pulver, das mit Wasser eingenommen wird.
All right, I try it at once!	Schön, gleich her damit!

Verlag von Julius Springer in Berlin N.

Hagers Handbuch der pharmaceutischen Praxis
für
Apotheker, Ärzte, Drogisten und Medizinalbeamte.
Unter Mitwirkung hervorragender Fachmänner
vollständig neu bearbeitet und herausgegeben von
B. Fischer und **C. Hartwich**
Breslau Zürich.
Zwei Bände. Mit zahlreichen in den Text gedruckten Holzschnitten.
Preis je M. 20.—, elegant in Halbleder gebunden je M. 22.50.
Auch in 20 Lieferungen zum Preise von je M. 2.— zu beziehen.

Neues pharmaceutisches Manual.
Herausgegeben von
Eugen Dietrich.
Mit in den Text gedruckten Holzschnitten.
Achte vermehrte Auflage.
In Moleskin geb. Preis M. 16.—, mit Schreibpapier durchschossen
und in Moleskin geb. M. 18.—.
Auch in 14 Lieferungen zum Preise von je M. 1.— zu beziehen.

Schule der Pharmacie
in 5 Bänden.
Herausgegeben von
Dr. J. Holfert, Prof. Dr. H. Thoms, Dr. E. Mylius, Dr. K. F. Jordan.

Band I: Praktischer Teil. Bearbeitet von Dr. E. Mylius. Mit 120 in den Text gedruckten Abbildungen. 2. Aufl. In Leinwand geb. Preis M. 4.—.
Band II: Chemischer Teil. Bearbeitet von Prof. Dr. H. Thoms. Mit 106 in den Text gedruckten Abbildungen. 3. Aufl. In Leinwand geb. Preis M. 7.—.
Band III: Physikalischer Teil. Bearbeitet von Dr. K. F. Jordan. Mit 142 in den Text gedruckten Abbildungen. 2. Aufl. In Leinwand geb. Preis M. 4.—.
Band IV: Botanischer Teil. Bearbeitet von Dr J. Holfert. Mit 465 in den Text gedruckten Abbildungen. 2. Aufl. In Leinwand geb. Preis M. 5.—.
Band V: Warenkunde. Bearbeitet von Prof. Dr. H. Thoms u. Dr. J. Holfert. Mit 194 in den Text gedruckten Abbild. 2. Aufl. In Leinw. geb. Pr. M. 6.—.

Jeder Band ist einzeln käuflich,

Pharmaceutische Übungspräparate.
Anleitung zur
Darstellung, Erkennung, Prüfung und stöchiometrischen Berechnung
von offizinellen chemisch-pharmaceutischen Präparaten.
Von **Dr. Max Biechele.**
Zweite Auflage unter der Presse.

Zu beziehen durch jede Buchhandlung.

Verlag von Julius Springer in Berlin N.

Spezialitäten und Geheimmittel
mit Angabe ihrer Zusammensetzung.
Eine Sammlung von Analysen, Gutachten und Literatur-Angaben.
Zusammengestellt von
Eduard Hahn und **Dr. J. Holfert.**
Fünfte, sehr vermehrte Auflage.
Preis M. 4.—, in Leinwand gebunden M. 5.—.

Pharmaceutische Synonyma
nebst ihren deutschen Bezeichnungen und ihren volkstümlichen Benennungen.
Ein Handbuch für Apotheker und Ärzte
zusammengestellt von
C. F. Schulze, Apotheker.
Preis M. 3.—, in Leinwand gebunden M. 4.—.

Volkstümliche Arzneimittelnamen.
Eine Sammlung der im
Volksmunde gebräuchlichen Benennungen der Apothekerwaren.
Von **Dr. J. Holfert.**
Dritte verbesserte und vermehrte Auflage,
bearbeitet von G. Arends.
Preis M. 3.—, in Leinwand gebunden M. 4.—.

Die kaufmännische Buchführung in der Apotheke,
nach bequemer und praktischer Methode
an der Hand eines Beispiels in instruktiver Weise dargestellt
von **Dr. W. Mayer,** Apotheker.
Dritte vermehrte Auflage.
Kart. Preis M. 1.40.

Kleiner Ratgeber für den Apothekenverkauf.
Von **Dr. E. Mylius,**
Besitzer der Engelapotheke in Leipzig.
Zweite vermehrte und verbesserte Auflage.
Preis M. 1.40.

Der Apotheker als Geschäftsmann.
Von **Dr. E. Mylius,**
Besitzer der Engelapotheke in Leipzig.
Preis M. 2.40.

Zu beziehen durch jede Buchhandlung.

MIX
Papier aus verantwortungsvollen Quellen
Paper from responsible sources
FSC® C105338

If you have any concerns about our products,
you can contact us on
ProductSafety@springernature.com

In case Publisher is established outside the EU,
the EU authorized representative is:
**Springer Nature Customer Service Center GmbH
Europaplatz 3, 69115 Heidelberg, Germany**

Printed by Libri Plureos GmbH
in Hamburg, Germany